RENTI JUTU

JIEPOUXUE

CAIHUI TUPU

人体局部解剖学
彩绘图谱

汪永锋　主编

甘肃科学技术出版社

图书在版编目（CIP）数据

人体局部解剖学彩绘图谱 / 汪永锋主编. -- 兰州：
甘肃科学技术出版社,2023.2（2023.9重印）
ISBN 978-7-5424-3036-6

Ⅰ．①人… Ⅱ．①汪… Ⅲ．①局部解剖学 - 图谱
Ⅳ．①R323-64

中国版本图书馆CIP数据核字（2023）第028387号

人体局部解剖学彩绘图谱

汪永锋　主编

责任编辑　李叶维
封面设计　雷们起

出　　版　甘肃科学技术出版社
社　　址　兰州市城关区曹家巷1号　730030
电　　话　0931-2131576（编辑部）　0931-8773237（发行部）

发　　行　甘肃科学技术出版社　　　印　刷　三河市铭诚印务有限公司
开　　本　787毫米×1092毫米　1/16　印　张　12.25　字　数　150千
版　　次　2023年3月第1版
印　　次　2023年9月第2次印刷
印　　数　2001~3050
书　　号　ISBN 978-7-5424-3036-6　　定　价　198.00元

前　言

　　《人体局部解剖学彩绘图谱》是在对人体系统解剖学的学习、研究基础上，将人体按部位分为头、颈、上肢、下肢、胸、腹、腰背、盆部与会阴八部分，分层次对人体局部的形态结构、器官毗邻关系等以彩色绘图形式进行表现和描述的形态学医学教学、研究材料，这是医学类学生和医务工作者步入临床学习、开展临床工作的工具书。

　　本图谱成书是对我校多年人体局部解剖学教学工作的总结性成果之一，是在我历年教学中使用线条图、黑白图、实物标本以及标本照片和彩色图谱教学的基础上，在 400 多张常用教学图中精选出 200 余张，对照局部解剖实际操作和制作的标本，绘制黑白线条图为蓝本，组织有多年解剖学教学、解剖标本制作和相当绘画水平的专业人员，采用工笔画技法，绘制而成。

在集中完成这些蓝本图及组织绘图的三年多时间里，有时虽然一天奔波千里，但仍坚持完成当天的审稿定稿，深夜方归；也有为了选择一种更好的表达方式，多方请教，反复思忖，夜不能寐，幡然顿悟的；得偿所愿，终于完成了《人体局部解剖学彩绘图谱》的全部绘制工作。虽呕心沥血，付梓不菲，但这对进一步总结、推进和逐步提升教学工作水平，启发学生学习，以致于在学生中组织开展人体解剖学图谱绘制竞赛活动，以及参加解剖学相关教材编写中提供有自主知识产权的图片等等奠定了良好基础，也必将为促进学习、教学、临床工作，推进学科建设创造更加有利条件。

在本书编写中，参阅了有关教材、图谱等大量的相关材料，在此对这些出版社和编者表示衷心感谢！并对所有参与绘制人员的辛勤付出表示诚挚的感谢！尤其要感谢我甘肃中医药大学解剖组胚教研室的同仁们，谢谢！很高兴我的研究生能积极主动参与校稿工作，这也很好地促进和丰富了他们的学习生活，教学相长，甚幸！

由于个人水平所限，本书编写错漏之处敬请批评指正，我们将再版时认真修正。

汪永锋

2017 年 10 月

目　录

第三章　上　肢 ··· 037

头部

第一章

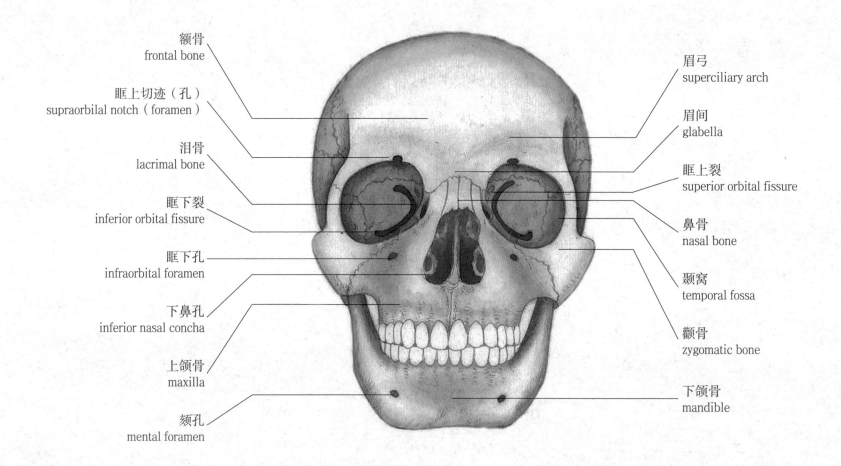

额骨
frontal bone

眶上切迹（孔）
supraorbilal notch（foramen）

泪骨
lacrimal bone

眶下裂
inferior orbital fissure

眶下孔
infraorbital foramen

下鼻孔
inferior nasal concha

上颌骨
maxilla

颏孔
mental foramen

眉弓
superciliary arch

眉间
glabella

眶上裂
superior orbital fissure

鼻骨
nasal bone

颞窝
temporal fossa

颧骨
zygomatic bone

下颌骨
mandible

图 1-1　颅的前面观
the skull（anterior view）

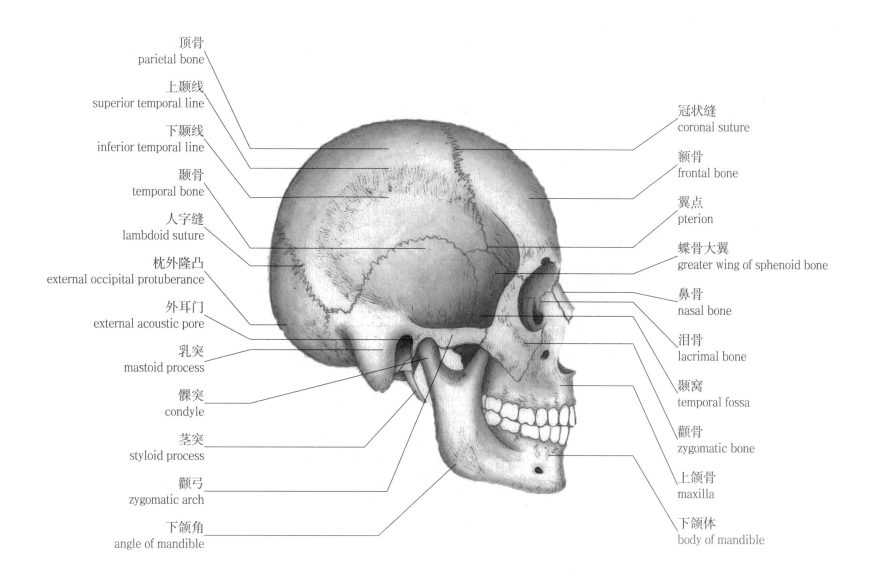

顶骨
parietal bone

上颞线
superior temporal line

下颞线
inferior temporal line

颞骨
temporal bone

人字缝
lambdoid suture

枕外隆凸
external occipital protuberance

外耳门
external acoustic pore

乳突
mastoid process

髁突
condyle

茎突
styloid process

颧弓
zygomatic arch

下颌角
angle of mandible

冠状缝
coronal suture

额骨
frontal bone

翼点
pterion

蝶骨大翼
greater wing of sphenoid bone

鼻骨
nasal bone

泪骨
lacrimal bone

颞窝
temporal fossa

颧骨
zygomatic bone

上颌骨
maxilla

下颌体
body of mandible

图 1-2 颅的侧面观
the sknll（lateral aspect）

滑车上动脉
supratrochlear artery

滑车上神经
supratrochlear nerve

眶上动脉
supraorbital artery

眶上神经
supraorbital nerve

内眦动、静脉
medial artery vein

面神经颧支
zygomatic branch of facial nerve

面神经颧支
zygomatic branch of facial nerve

面横动脉
transverse facial artery

腮腺管
parotid duct

面神经颊支
buccal branch of facial nerve

面静脉
facial vein

面神经下颌缘支
marginal mandibular branch of facial nerve

耳后动静脉
posterior auricular artery vein

耳颞神经
ciculotemporal nerve

枕大神经
greater occipital nerve

颞浅静脉
srperficial temporal vein

枕动、静脉
occipital vein

腮腺
parotid

枕小神经
lesser occipital nerve

咬肌
masseter

颈外静脉
external jugular vein

耳大神经
great auricular never

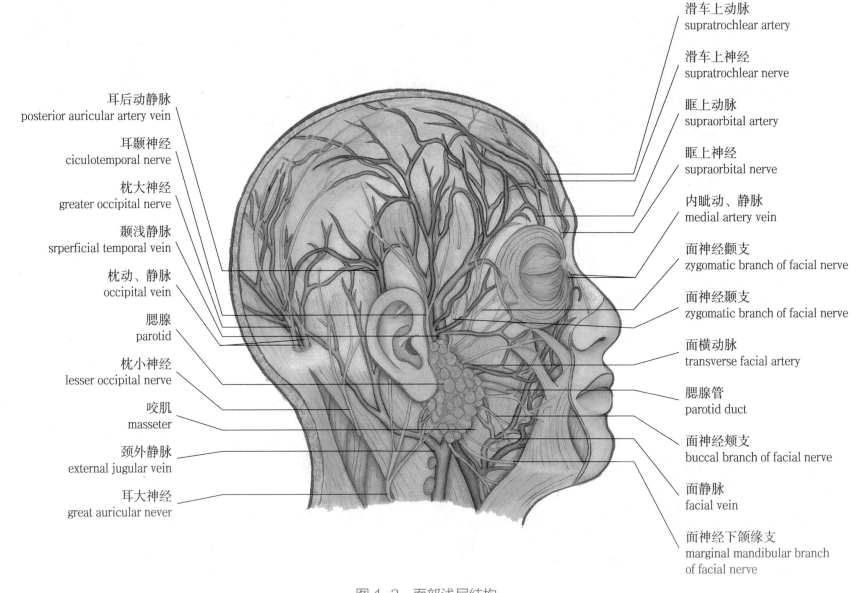

图 1-3　面部浅层结构
the face（lateral aspect）

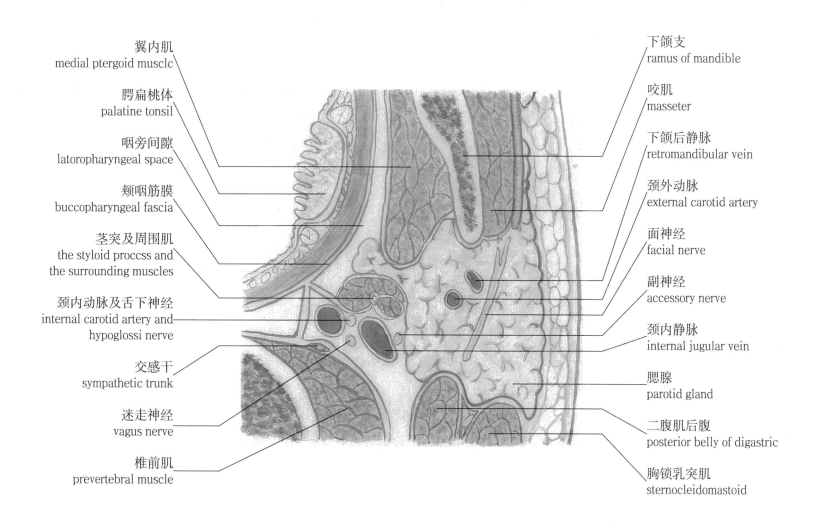

翼内肌
medial ptergoid musclc

腭扁桃体
palatine tonsil

咽旁间隙
latoropharyngeal space

颊咽筋膜
buccopharyngeal fascia

茎突及周围肌
the styloid proccss and
the surrounding muscles

颈内动脉及舌下神经
internal carotid artery and
hypoglossi nerve

交感干
sympathetic trunk

迷走神经
vagus nerve

椎前肌
prevertebral muscle

下颌支
ramus of mandible

咬肌
masseter

下颌后静脉
retromandibular vein

颈外动脉
external carotid artery

面神经
facial nerve

副神经
accessory nerve

颈内静脉
internal jugular vein

腮腺
parotid gland

二腹肌后腹
posterior belly of digastric

胸锁乳突肌
sternocleidomastoid

图 1-4　腮腺和面侧区水平断面（右侧、上面观）
horizontal section of the parotid gland and face（right superior view）

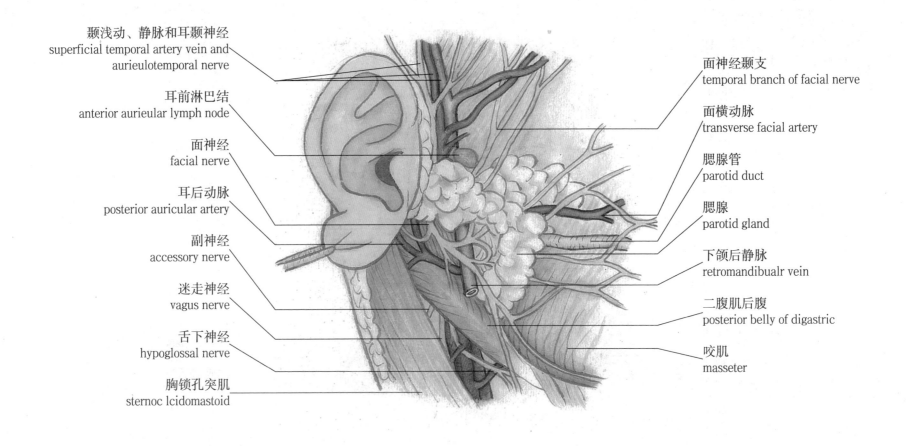

颞浅动、静脉和耳颞神经
superficial temporal artery vein and aurieulotemporal nerve

耳前淋巴结
anterior aurieular lymph node

面神经
facial nerve

耳后动脉
posterior auricular artery

副神经
accessory nerve

迷走神经
vagus nerve

舌下神经
hypoglossal nerve

胸锁孔突肌
sternoc lcidomastoid

面神经颞支
temporal branch of facial nerve

面横动脉
transverse facial artery

腮腺管
parotid duct

腮腺
parotid gland

下颌后静脉
retromandibualr vein

二腹肌后腹
posterior belly of digastric

咬肌
masseter

图 1-5 腮腺及穿经腮腺的血管、神经
Parotid gland and structure passes through the parotid gland

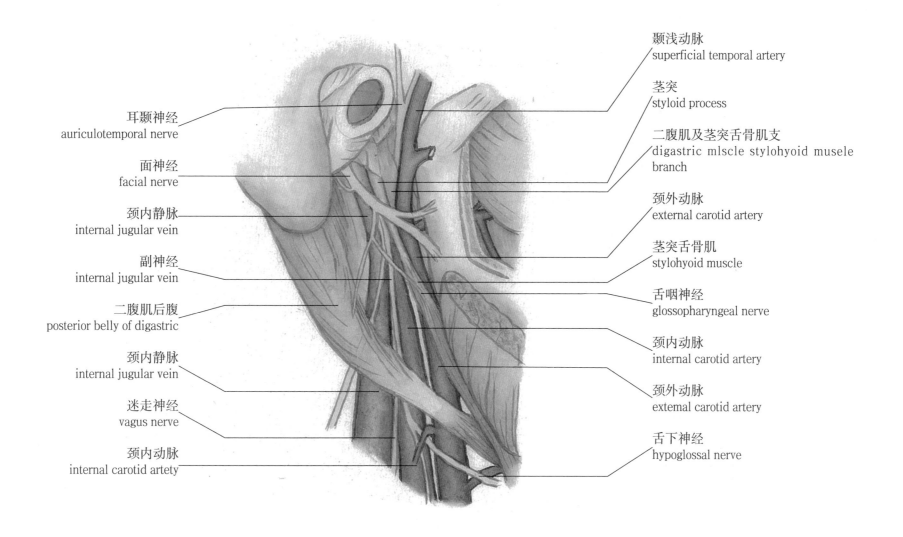

颞浅动脉
superficial temporal artery

茎突
styloid process

二腹肌及茎突舌骨肌支
digastric mlscle stylohyoid musele branch

颈外动脉
external carotid artery

茎突舌骨肌
stylohyoid muscle

舌咽神经
glossopharyngeal nerve

颈内动脉
internal carotid artery

颈外动脉
extemal carotid artery

舌下神经
hypoglossal nerve

耳颞神经
auriculotemporal nerve

面神经
facial nerve

颈内静脉
internal jugular vein

副神经
internal jugular vein

二腹肌后腹
posterior belly of digastric

颈内静脉
internal jugular vein

迷走神经
vagus nerve

颈内动脉
internal carotid artety

图 1-6 腮腺深面的结构

stucture of the deep surface of the parotid gland

耳颞神经
auriculotemporal nerve

颞浅动脉
superficial temporal artery

颞浅静脉
superficial temporal vein

咬肌神经
masseteric nerve

上颌动脉
maxillary artery

面神经
facial nerve

下牙槽神经
inferior alveolar nerve

下牙槽动脉
inferior alveolar artery

颈外动脉
external carotid artery

下颌后静脉
retromandibular vein

咬肌
masseter

颞肌
temporalis

上颌动脉
maxillary artery

翼外肌
lateral pterygoid mujscle

颊动脉
buccal artery

颊神经
buccal nerve

翼内肌
medial pterygoid muscle

舌神经
lingual nerve

颊肌
buccinator

面静脉
facial vein

面动脉
facial artety

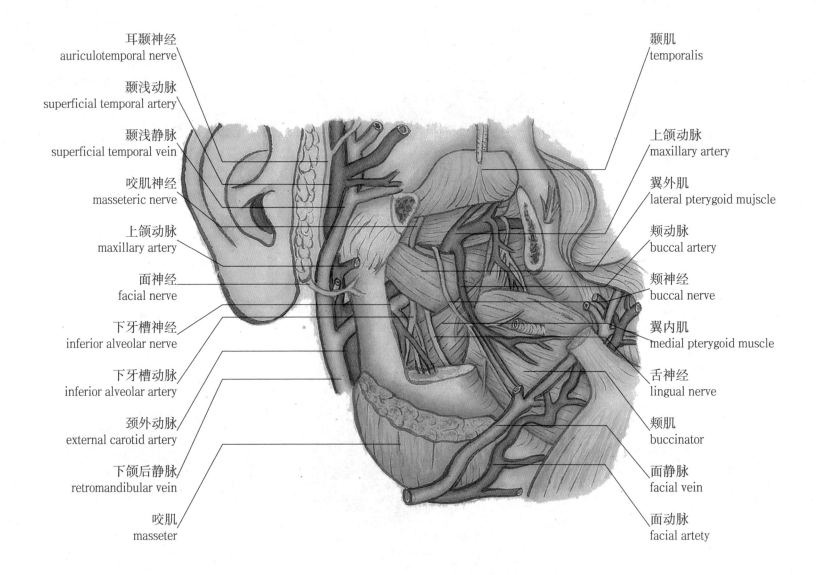

图 1-7　面侧深区的血管和神经（浅部）

Vessles and nerves of the deep layer of the face（shallow view）

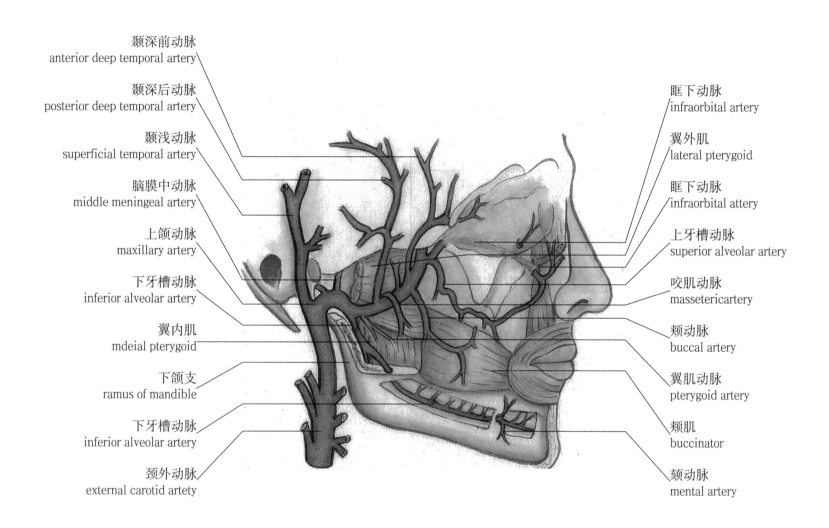

颞深前动脉
anterior deep temporal artery

颞深后动脉
posterior deep temporal artery

颞浅动脉
superficial temporal artery

脑膜中动脉
middle meningeal artery

上颌动脉
maxillary artery

下牙槽动脉
inferior alveolar artery

翼内肌
mdeial pterygoid

下颌支
ramus of mandible

下牙槽动脉
inferior alveolar artery

颈外动脉
external carotid artety

眶下动脉
infraorbital artery

翼外肌
lateral pterygoid

眶下动脉
infraorbital attery

上牙槽动脉
superior alveolar artery

咬肌动脉
masstericartery

颊动脉
buccal artery

翼肌动脉
pterygoid artery

颊肌
buccinator

颏动脉
mental artery

图 1-8 上颌动脉的行程及分支
maxillary artery and its branches

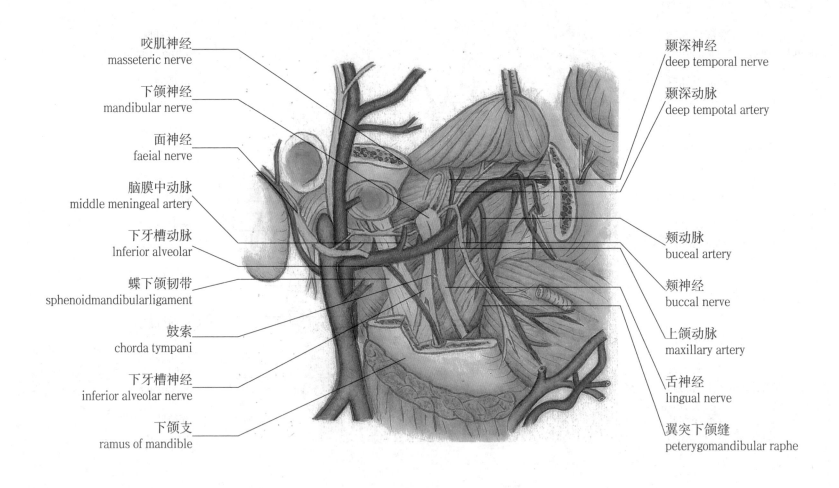

咬肌神经
masseteric nerve

下颌神经
mandibular nerve

面神经
faeial nerve

脑膜中动脉
middle meningeal artery

下牙槽动脉
lnferior alveolar

蝶下颌韧带
sphenoidmandibularligament

鼓索
chorda tympani

下牙槽神经
inferior alveolar nerve

下颌支
ramus of mandible

颞深神经
deep temporal nerve

颞深动脉
deep tempotal artery

颊动脉
buceal artery

颊神经
buccal nerve

上颌动脉
maxillary artery

舌神经
lingual nerve

翼突下颌缝
peterygomandibular raphe

图 1-9　面侧深区的血管和神经（深部）

Blood vessels and nerves of the deep layer of the face（deep view）

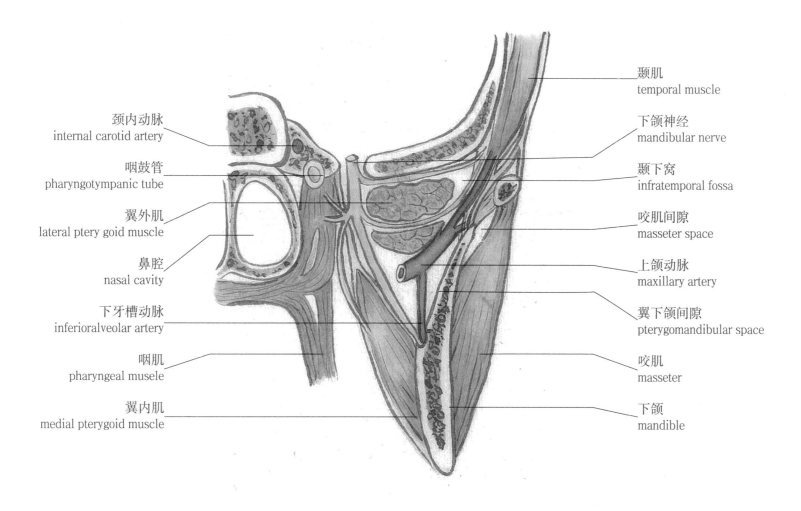

颞肌
temporal muscle

下颌神经
mandibular nerve

颈内动脉
internal carotid artery

颞下窝
infratemporal fossa

咽鼓管
pharyngotympanic tube

翼外肌
lateral ptery goid muscle

咬肌间隙
masseter space

鼻腔
nasal cavity

上颌动脉
maxillary artery

下牙槽动脉
inferioralveolar artery

翼下颌间隙
pterygomandibular space

咽肌
pharyngeal musele

咬肌
masseter

翼内肌
medial pterygoid muscle

下颌
mandible

图 1-10 面部间隙（冠状面）
space of the face（coronal sectio）

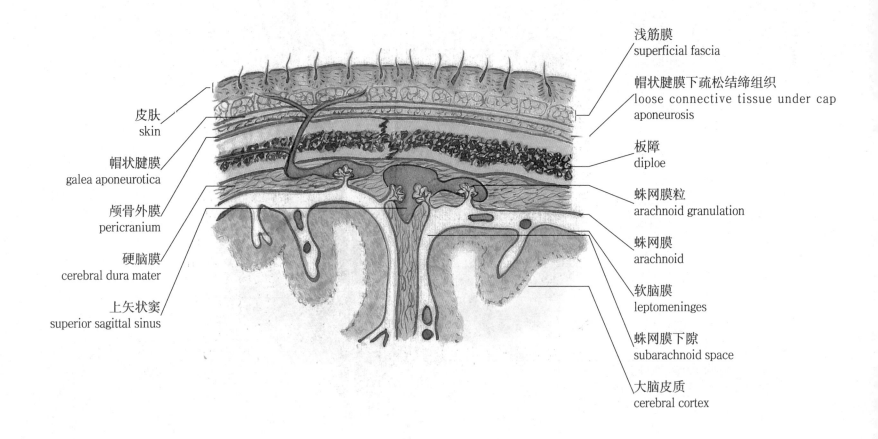

皮肤
skin

帽状腱膜
galea aponeurotica

颅骨外膜
pericranium

硬脑膜
cerebral dura mater

上矢状窦
superior sagittal sinus

浅筋膜
superficial fascia

帽状腱膜下疏松结缔组织
loose connective tissue under cap
aponeurosis

板障
diploe

蛛网膜粒
arachnoid granulation

蛛网膜
arachnoid

软脑膜
leptomeninges

蛛网膜下隙
subarachnoid space

大脑皮质
cerebral cortex

图 1-11 颅顶层次（额状面）
Parietal structure（coronal aspect）

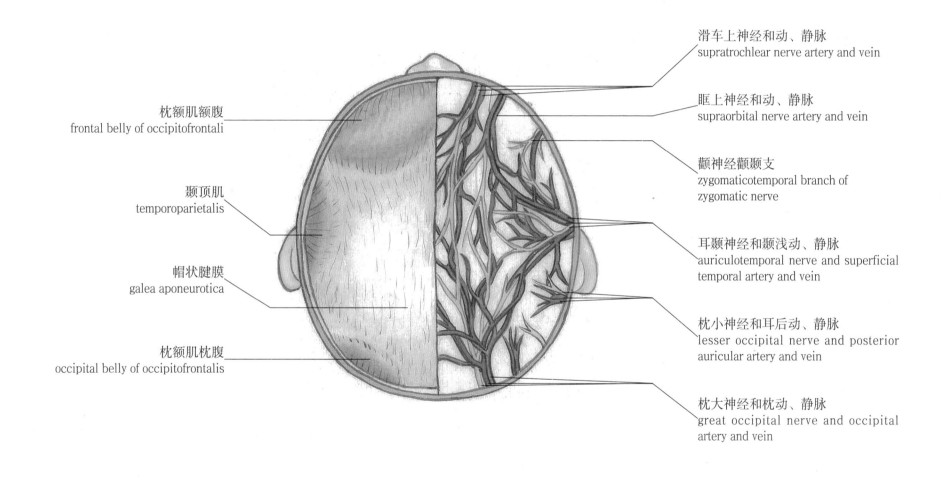

滑车上神经和动、静脉
supratrochlear nerve artery and vein

眶上神经和动、静脉
supraorbital nerve artery and vein

颧神经颧颞支
zygomaticotemporal branch of
zygomatic nerve

耳颞神经和颞浅动、静脉
auriculotemporal nerve and superficial
temporal artery and vein

枕小神经和耳后动、静脉
lesser occipital nerve and posterior
auricular artery and vein

枕大神经和枕动、静脉
great occipital nerve and occipital
artery and vein

枕额肌额腹
frontal belly of occipitofrontali

颞顶肌
temporoparietalis

帽状腱膜
galea aponeurotica

枕额肌枕腹
occipital belly of occipitofrontalis

图 1-12 颅顶部血管、神经
Parietal blood vessels and nerves

颈部

第二章

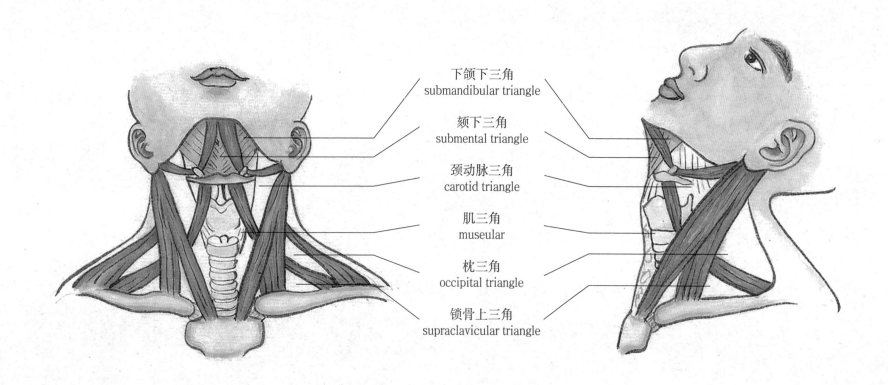

下颌下三角
submandibular triangle

颏下三角
submental triangle

颈动脉三角
carotid triangle

肌三角
museular

枕三角
occipital triangle

锁骨上三角
supraclavicular triangle

图 2-1　颈部分区

Borders and subdivisions of the neck

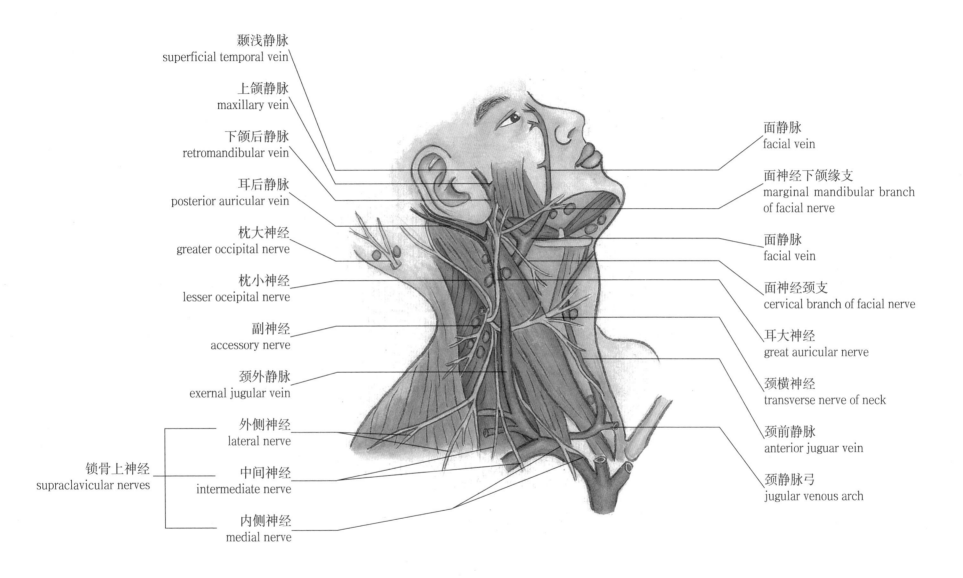

颞浅静脉
superficial temporal vein

上颌静脉
maxillary vein

下颌后静脉
retromandibular vein

耳后静脉
posterior auricular vein

枕大神经
greater occipital nerve

枕小神经
lesser oceipital nerve

副神经
accessory nerve

颈外静脉
exernal jugular vein

锁骨上神经
supraclavicular nerves

外侧神经
lateral nerve

中间神经
intermediate nerve

内侧神经
medial nerve

面静脉
facial vein

面神经下颌缘支
marginal mandibular branch
of facial nerve

面静脉
facial vein

面神经颈支
cervical branch of facial nerve

耳大神经
great auricular nerve

颈横神经
transverse nerve of neck

颈前静脉
anterior juguar vein

颈静脉弓
jugular venous arch

图 2-2 颈部浅层结构
Superficial structure of the neck

气管前间隙
pretracheal space

甲状腺假被膜
false thyroid capsule

甲状腺真被膜
true thyroid capsule

颈动脉鞘
carotid sheath

交感干
cervical svmpathetic trunk

椎前筋膜
prevertebral fascia

膈神经
phrenic nerve

颈前静脉
anterior jugular vein

颈深筋膜浅层
suerfieial layer of deep cervical fascia

舌骨下肌群
infrahyoid muscles

胸锁乳突肌
sternocleidomastoid muscle

咽后间隙
retrophar yngeal space

椎前间隙
prevertebral space

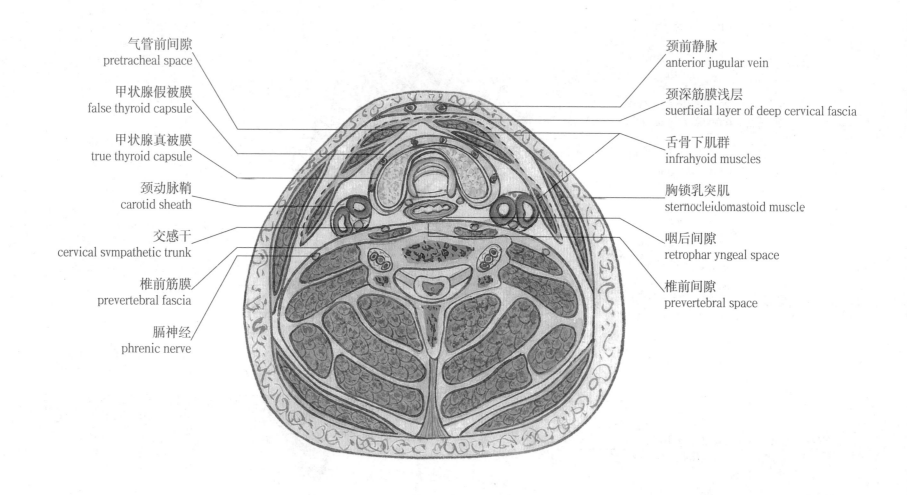

图 2-3　颈筋膜（横切面）
Cervical fascia（horizontal section）

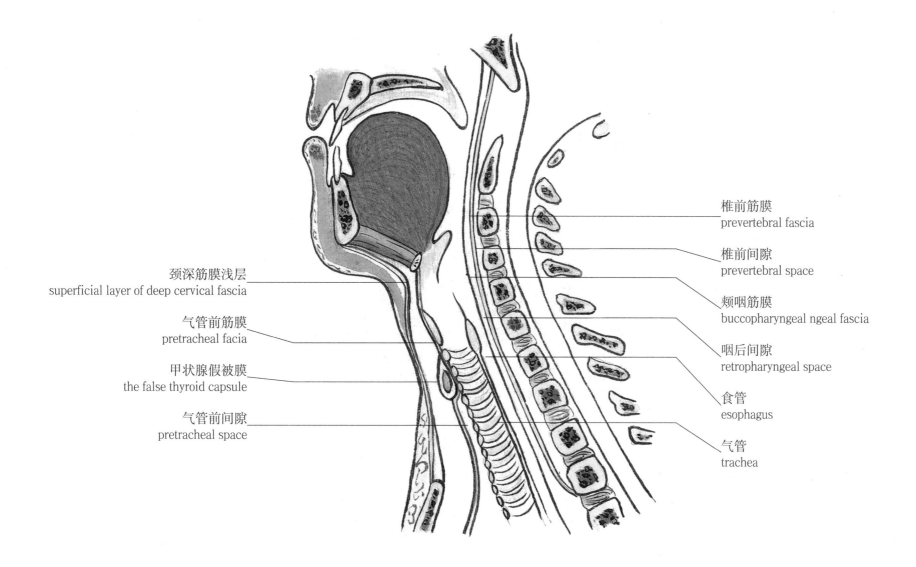

颈深筋膜浅层
superficial layer of deep cervical fascia

气管前筋膜
pretracheal facia

甲状腺假被膜
the false thyroid capsule

气管前间隙
pretracheal space

椎前筋膜
prevertebral fascia

椎前间隙
prevertebral space

颊咽筋膜
buccopharyngeal ngeal fascia

咽后间隙
retropharyngeal space

食管
esophagus

气管
trachea

图 2-4 颈筋膜（正中矢状面）
Cervical fascia（mdeian sagittal section）

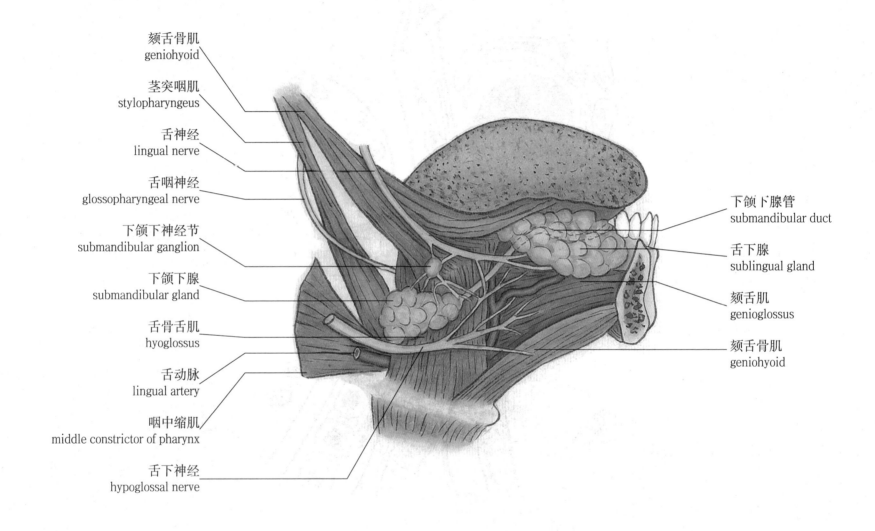

颏舌骨肌
geniohyoid

茎突咽肌
stylopharyngeus

舌神经
lingual nerve

舌咽神经
glossopharyngeal nerve

下颌下神经节
submandibular ganglion

下颌下腺
submandibular gland

舌骨舌肌
hyoglossus

舌动脉
lingual artery

咽中缩肌
middle constrictor of pharynx

舌下神经
hypoglossal nerve

下颌下腺管
submandibular duct

舌下腺
sublingual gland

颏舌肌
genioglossus

颏舌骨肌
geniohyoid

图 2-5　下颌下三角内容
Submandibular triangle structure

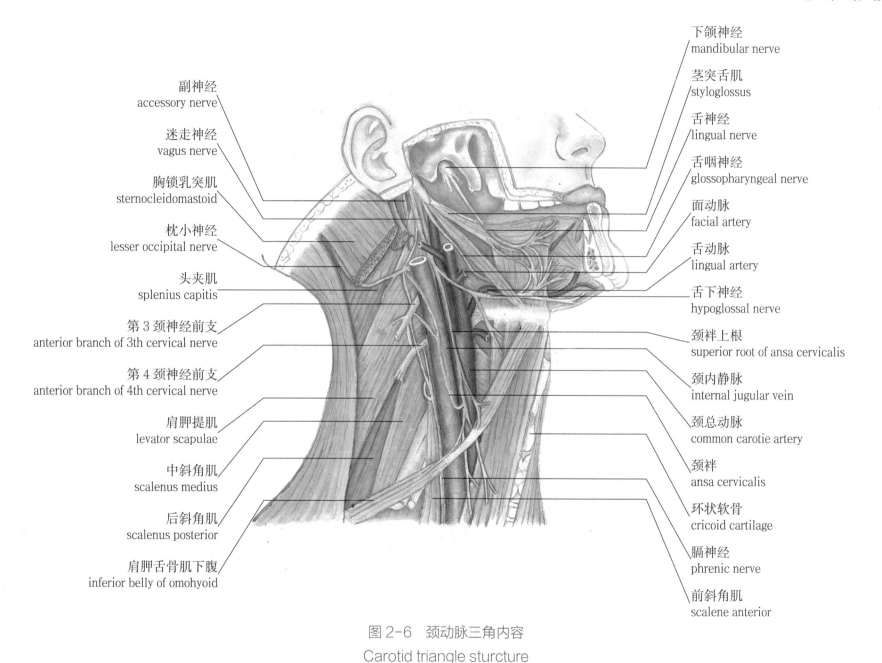

副神经
accessory nerve

迷走神经
vagus nerve

胸锁乳突肌
sternocleidomastoid

枕小神经
lesser occipital nerve

头夹肌
splenius capitis

第 3 颈神经前支
anterior branch of 3th cervical nerve

第 4 颈神经前支
anterior branch of 4th cervical nerve

肩胛提肌
levator scapulae

中斜角肌
scalenus medius

后斜角肌
scalenus posterior

肩胛舌骨肌下腹
inferior belly of omohyoid

下颌神经
mandibular nerve

茎突舌肌
styloglossus

舌神经
lingual nerve

舌咽神经
glossopharyngeal nerve

面动脉
facial artery

舌动脉
lingual artery

舌下神经
hypoglossal nerve

颈袢上根
superior root of ansa cervicalis

颈内静脉
internal jugular vein

颈总动脉
common carotie artery

颈袢
ansa cervicalis

环状软骨
cricoid cartilage

膈神经
phrenic nerve

前斜角肌
scalene anterior

图 2-6 颈动脉三角内容
Carotid triangle sturcture

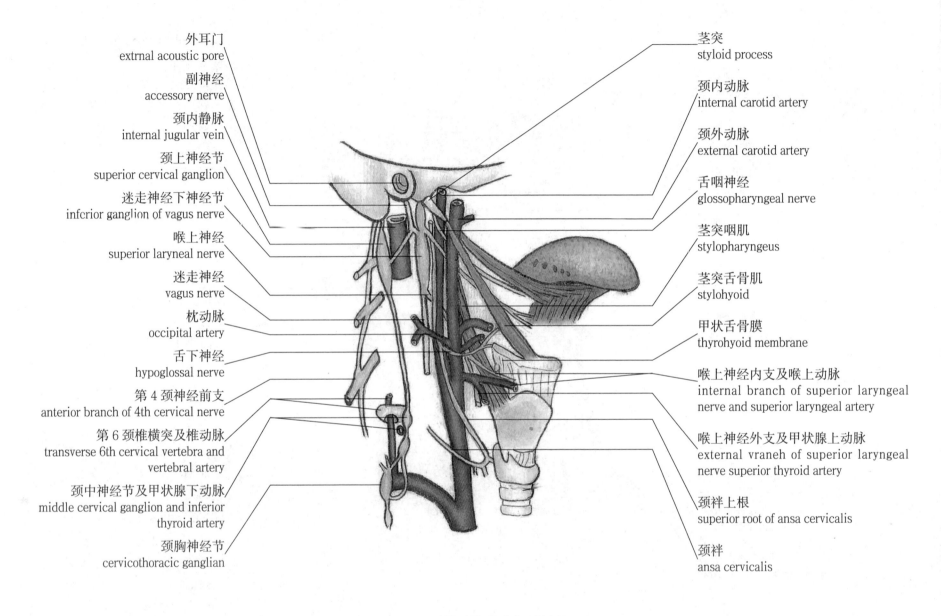

外耳门
extrnal acoustic pore

副神经
accessory nerve

颈内静脉
internal jugular vein

颈上神经节
superior cervical ganglion

迷走神经下神经节
infcrior ganglion of vagus nerve

喉上神经
superior laryneal nerve

迷走神经
vagus nerve

枕动脉
occipital artery

舌下神经
hypoglossal nerve

第 4 颈神经前支
anterior branch of 4th cervical nerve

第 6 颈椎横突及椎动脉
transverse 6th cervical vertebra and
vertebral artery

颈中神经节及甲状腺下动脉
middle cervical ganglion and inferior
thyroid artery

颈胸神经节
cervicothoracic ganglian

茎突
styloid process

颈内动脉
internal carotid artery

颈外动脉
external carotid artery

舌咽神经
glossopharyngeal nerve

茎突咽肌
stylopharyngeus

茎突舌骨肌
stylohyoid

甲状舌骨膜
thyrohyoid membrane

喉上神经内支及喉上动脉
internal branch of superior laryngeal
nerve and superior laryngeal artery

喉上神经外支及甲状腺上动脉
external vraneh of superior laryngeal
nerve superior thyroid artery

颈袢上根
superior root of ansa cervicalis

颈袢
ansa cervicalis

图 2-7　颈总动脉分支与脑神经
Branches of common carotid artery and cranial nerves

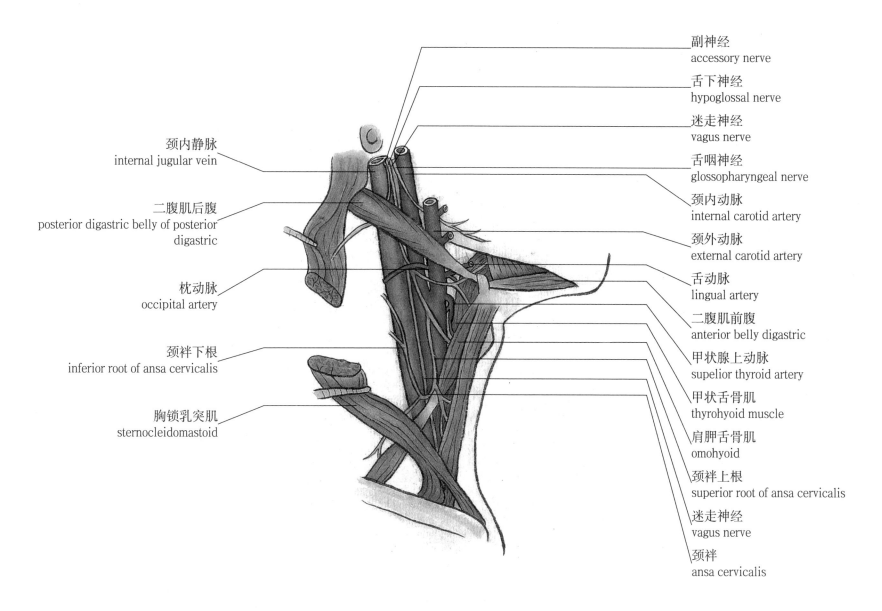

颈内静脉
internal jugular vein

二腹肌后腹
posterior digastric belly of posterior digastric

枕动脉
occipital artery

颈袢下根
inferior root of ansa cervicalis

胸锁乳突肌
sternocleidomastoid

副神经
accessory nerve

舌下神经
hypoglossal nerve

迷走神经
vagus nerve

舌咽神经
glossopharyngeal nerve

颈内动脉
internal carotid artery

颈外动脉
external carotid artery

舌动脉
lingual artery

二腹肌前腹
anterior belly digastric

甲状腺上动脉
supelior thyroid artery

甲状舌骨肌
thyrohyoid muscle

肩胛舌骨肌
omohyoid

颈袢上根
superior root of ansa cervicalis

迷走神经
vagus nerve

颈袢
ansa cervicalis

图 2-8 二腹肌后腹的毗邻
Posterior belly of digastric and its relations

颈前静脉
anterior jugular vein

颏下静脉
submental vein

下颌下腺
submandibular gland

下颌后静脉
retromandibular vein

茎突舌骨肌
stylohyoid

面静脉
facial vein

颈内静脉
internal jugular vein

甲状腺上静脉
superior thyroid vein

颈外静脉
extemal jugular vein

颈总动脉
common carotid artery

胸锁乳突肌
sternocleidomastoid

颈静脉弓
jugular venous arch

甲状腺下静脉
inferior thyroid vein

颏下静脉
submental vein

面动脉
facial artery

面静脉
facial vein

舌下神经
hypoglossal nerve

腮腺
parotid gland

面静脉
facial vein

颈外静脉
external jugular vein

甲状软骨
thyroid cartilage

甲状腺上静脉
superior thyroid vein

颈袢
ansa cervical

颈内静脉
internal jugular vein

甲状腺峡
lsthmus of thyroid gland

颈外静脉
external jugular vein

颈前静脉
anterior jugualr

肩胛舌骨肌
omohyoid muscle

胸锁乳突肌
sternocleidomastoid

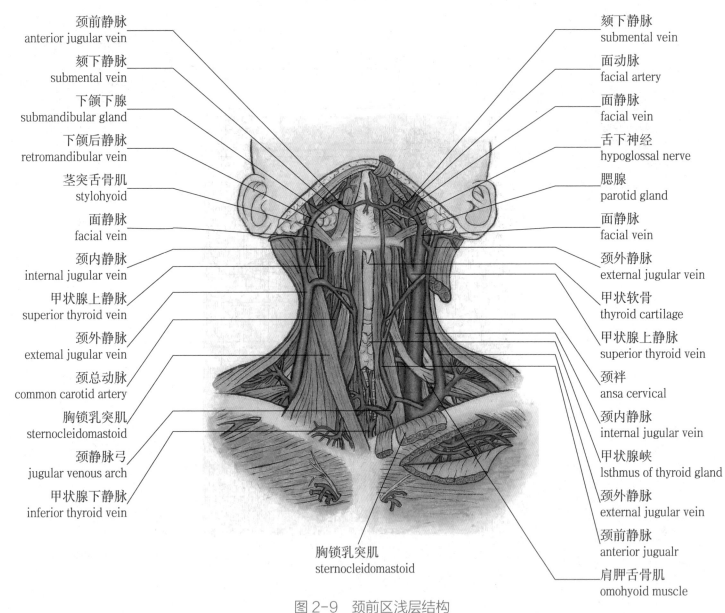

图 2-9　颈前区浅层结构
Superficial structure of anterior triangle of the neck

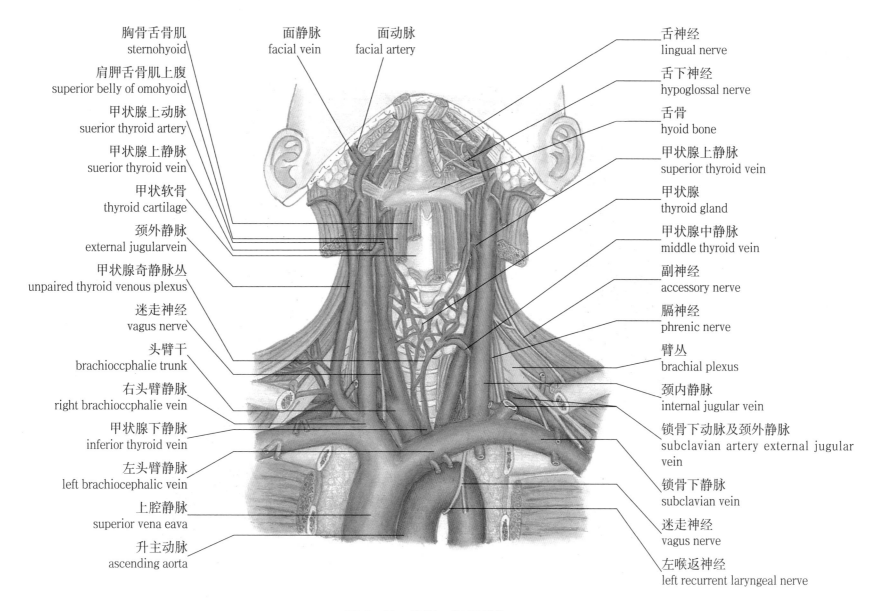

胸骨舌骨肌
sternohyoid

肩胛舌骨肌上腹
superior belly of omohyoid

甲状腺上动脉
suerior thyroid artery

甲状腺上静脉
suerior thyroid vein

甲状软骨
thyroid cartilage

颈外静脉
external jugularvein

甲状腺奇静脉丛
unpaired thyroid venous plexus

迷走神经
vagus nerve

头臂干
brachioccphalie trunk

右头臂静脉
right brachioccphalie vein

甲状腺下静脉
inferior thyroid vein

左头臂静脉
left brachiocephalic vein

上腔静脉
superior vena eava

升主动脉
ascending aorta

面静脉
facial vein

面动脉
facial artery

舌神经
lingual nerve

舌下神经
hypoglossal nerve

舌骨
hyoid bone

甲状腺上静脉
superior thyroid vein

甲状腺
thyroid gland

甲状腺中静脉
middle thyroid vein

副神经
accessory nerve

膈神经
phrenic nerve

臂丛
brachial plexus

颈内静脉
internal jugular vein

锁骨下动脉及颈外静脉
subclavian artery external jugular vein

锁骨下静脉
subclavian vein

迷走神经
vagus nerve

左喉返神经
left recurrent laryngeal nerve

图 2-10　颈前区深层结构
Deep structure of anterior triangle of the neck

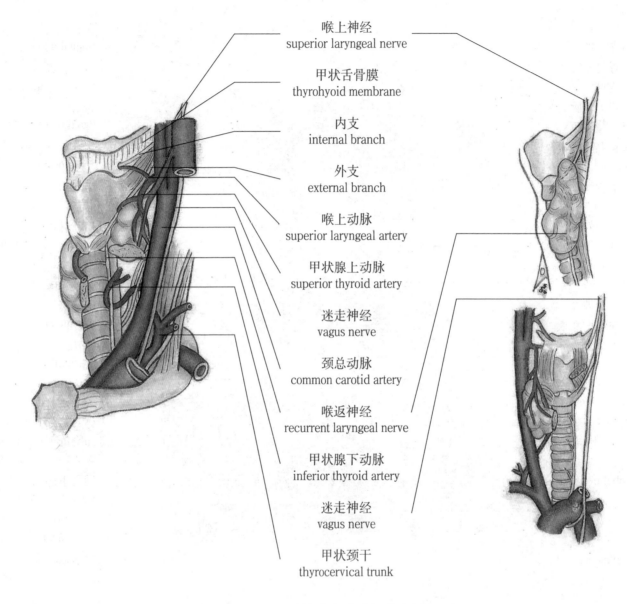

喉上神经
superior laryngeal nerve

甲状舌骨膜
thyrohyoid membrane

内支
internal branch

外支
external branch

喉上动脉
superior laryngeal artery

甲状腺上动脉
superior thyroid artery

迷走神经
vagus nerve

颈总动脉
common carotid artery

喉返神经
recurrent laryngeal nerve

甲状腺下动脉
inferior thyroid artery

迷走神经
vagus nerve

甲状颈干
thyrocervical trunk

图 2-11　甲状腺上动脉与喉上神经
Superior thyroid artery and superior laryngeal nerve

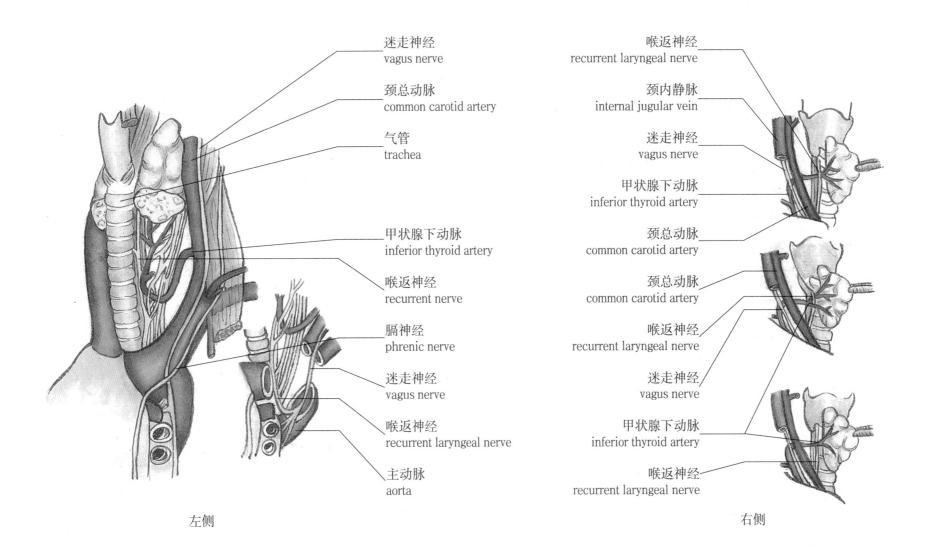

迷走神经
vagus nerve

颈总动脉
common carotid artery

气管
trachea

甲状腺下动脉
inferior thyroid artery

喉返神经
recurrent nerve

膈神经
phrenic nerve

迷走神经
vagus nerve

喉返神经
recurrent laryngeal nerve

主动脉
aorta

喉返神经
recurrent laryngeal nerve

颈内静脉
internal jugular vein

迷走神经
vagus nerve

甲状腺下动脉
inferior thyroid artery

颈总动脉
common carotid artery

颈总动脉
common carotid artery

喉返神经
recurrent laryngeal nerve

迷走神经
vagus nerve

甲状腺下动脉
inferior thyroid artery

喉返神经
recurrent laryngeal nerve

左侧

右侧

图 2-12　甲状腺下动脉与喉返神经
Inferior thyroid artery and recurrent laryngeal nerve

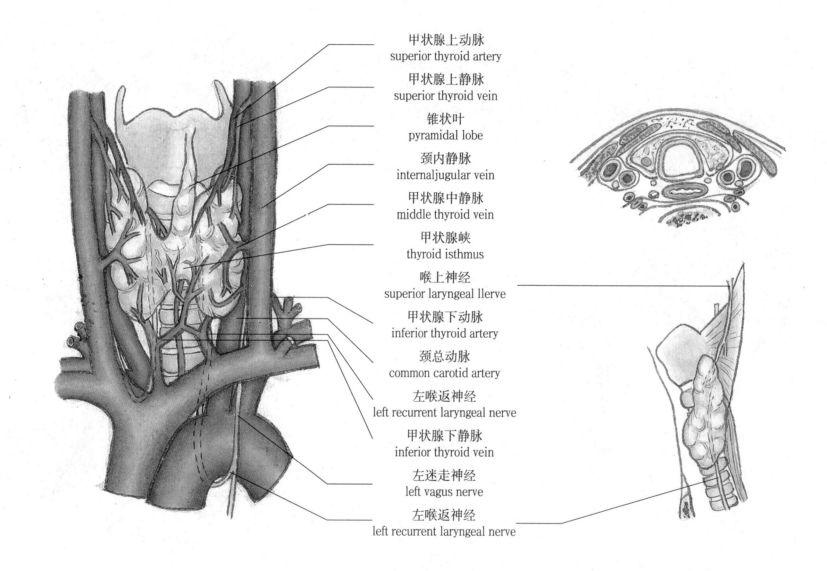

甲状腺上动脉
superior thyroid artery

甲状腺上静脉
superior thyroid vein

锥状叶
pyramidal lobe

颈内静脉
internaljugular vein

甲状腺中静脉
middle thyroid vein

甲状腺峡
thyroid isthmus

喉上神经
superior laryngeal llerve

甲状腺下动脉
inferior thyroid artery

颈总动脉
common carotid artery

左喉返神经
left recurrent laryngeal nerve

甲状腺下静脉
inferior thyroid vein

左迷走神经
left vagus nerve

左喉返神经
left recurrent laryngeal nerve

图 2-13 甲状腺的静脉
Vasculature of the thyroid gland

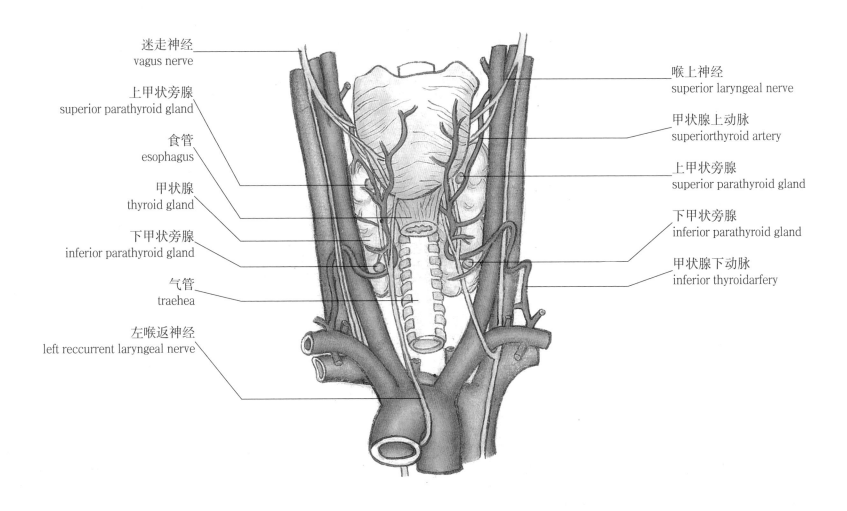

迷走神经
vagus nerve

上甲状旁腺
superior parathyroid gland

食管
esophagus

甲状腺
thyroid gland

下甲状旁腺
inferior parathyroid gland

气管
traehea

左喉返神经
left reccurrent laryngeal nerve

喉上神经
superior laryngeal nerve

甲状腺上动脉
superiorthyroid artery

上甲状旁腺
superior parathyroid gland

下甲状旁腺
inferior parathyroid gland

甲状腺下动脉
inferior thyroidarfery

图 2-14 甲状腺旁腺
Parathyroid gland

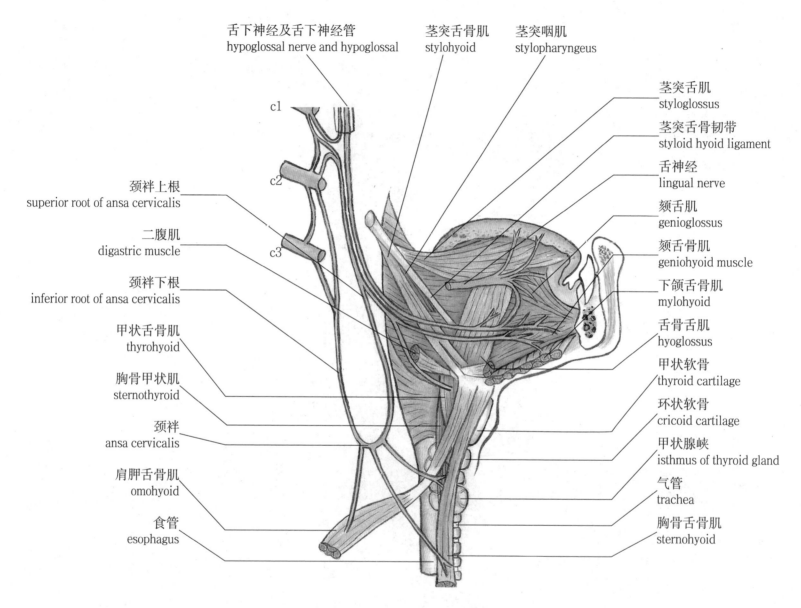

舌下神经及舌下神经管
hypoglossal nerve and hypoglossal

茎突舌骨肌
stylohyoid

茎突咽肌
stylopharyngeus

茎突舌肌
styloglossus

茎突舌骨韧带
styloid hyoid ligament

舌神经
lingual nerve

颏舌肌
genioglossus

颏舌骨肌
geniohyoid muscle

下颌舌骨肌
mylohyoid

舌骨舌肌
hyoglossus

甲状软骨
thyroid cartilage

环状软骨
cricoid cartilage

甲状腺峡
isthmus of thyroid gland

气管
trachea

胸骨舌骨肌
sternohyoid

c1

c2

c3

颈袢上根
superior root of ansa cervicalis

二腹肌
digastric muscle

颈袢下根
inferior root of ansa cervicalis

甲状舌骨肌
thyrohyoid

胸骨甲状肌
sternothyroid

颈袢
ansa cervicalis

肩胛舌骨肌
omohyoid

食管
esophagus

图 2-15 颈袢及支配的肌
Ansa cervicalis and innervation of muscle

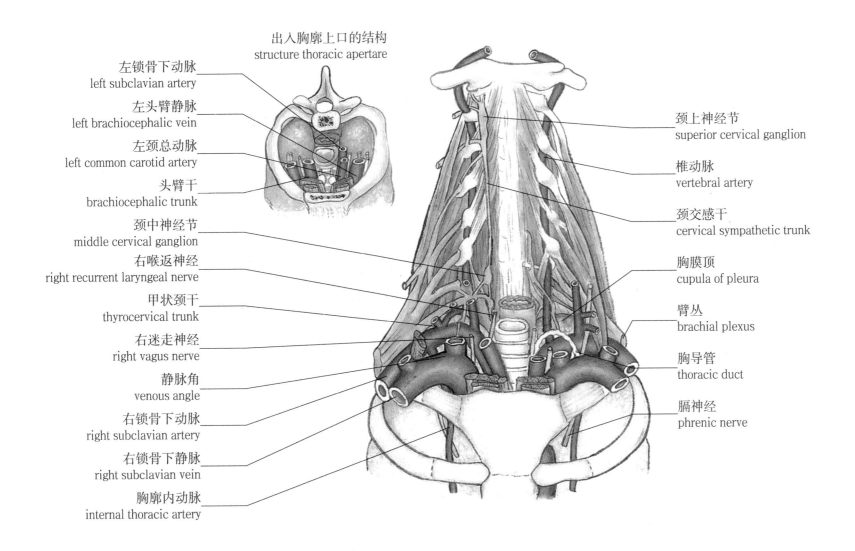

左锁骨下动脉
left subclavian artery

出入胸廓上口的结构
structure thoracic apertare

左头臂静脉
left brachiocephalic vein

左颈总动脉
left common carotid artery

头臂干
brachiocephalic trunk

颈中神经节
middle cervical ganglion

右喉返神经
right recurrent laryngeal nerve

甲状颈干
thyrocervical trunk

右迷走神经
right vagus nerve

静脉角
venous angle

右锁骨下动脉
right subclavian artery

右锁骨下静脉
right subclavian vein

胸廓内动脉
internal thoracic artery

颈上神经节
superior cervical ganglion

椎动脉
vertebral artery

颈交感干
cervical sympathetic trunk

胸膜顶
cupula of pleura

臂丛
brachial plexus

胸导管
thoracic duct

膈神经
phrenic nerve

图 2-16 颈根部
structure of the root of neck

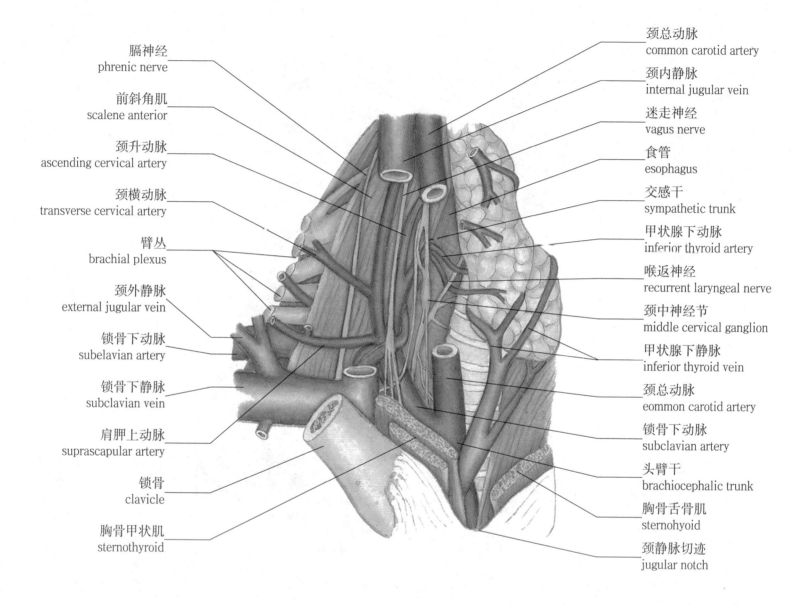

膈神经
phrenic nerve

前斜角肌
scalene anterior

颈升动脉
ascending cervical artery

颈横动脉
transverse cervical artery

臂丛
brachial plexus

颈外静脉
external jugular vein

锁骨下动脉
subelavian artery

锁骨下静脉
subclavian vein

肩胛上动脉
suprascapular artery

锁骨
clavicle

胸骨甲状肌
sternothyroid

颈总动脉
common carotid artery

颈内静脉
internal jugular vein

迷走神经
vagus nerve

食管
esophagus

交感干
sympathetic trunk

甲状腺下动脉
inferior thyroid artery

喉返神经
recurrent laryngeal nerve

颈中神经节
middle cervical ganglion

甲状腺下静脉
inferior thyroid vein

颈总动脉
eommon carotid artery

锁骨下动脉
subclavian artery

头臂干
brachiocephalic trunk

胸骨舌骨肌
sternohyoid

颈静脉切迹
jugular notch

图 2-17　前斜角肌的毗邻
Neighbourhood of scalene anterior

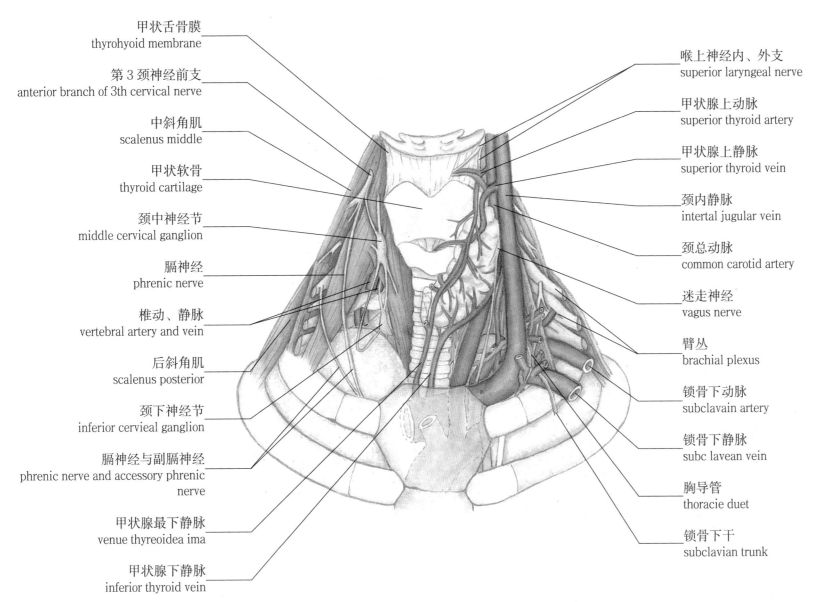

甲状舌骨膜
thyrohyoid membrane

第 3 颈神经前支
anterior branch of 3th cervical nerve

中斜角肌
scalenus middle

甲状软骨
thyroid cartilage

颈中神经节
middle cervical ganglion

膈神经
phrenic nerve

椎动、静脉
vertebral artery and vein

后斜角肌
scalenus posterior

颈下神经节
inferior cervieal ganglion

膈神经与副膈神经
phrenic nerve and accessory phrenic nerve

甲状腺最下静脉
venue thyreoidea ima

甲状腺下静脉
inferior thyroid vein

喉上神经内、外支
superior laryngeal nerve

甲状腺上动脉
superior thyroid artery

甲状腺上静脉
superior thyroid vein

颈内静脉
intertal jugular vein

颈总动脉
common carotid artery

迷走神经
vagus nerve

臂丛
brachial plexus

锁骨下动脉
subclavain artery

锁骨下静脉
subc lavean vein

胸导管
thoracie duet

锁骨下干
subclavian trunk

图 2-18 椎动脉三角及其内容
Vertebral artery triangle and its contents

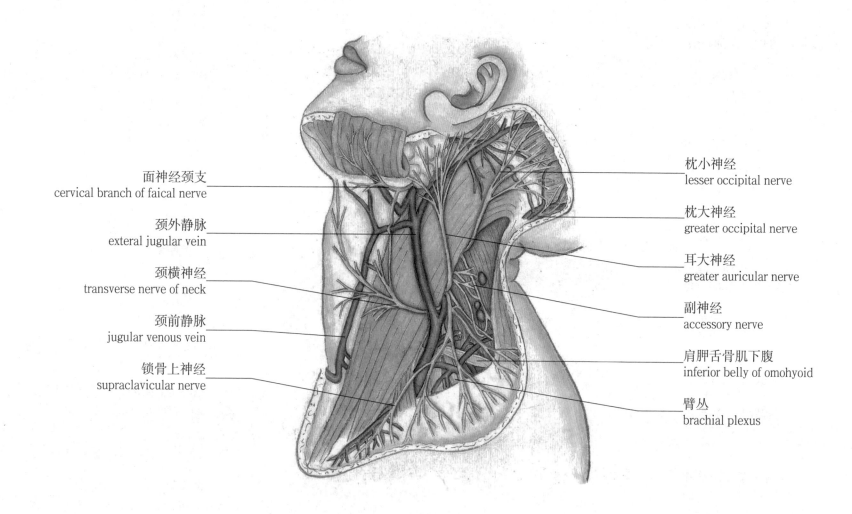

面神经颈支
cervical branch of faical nerve

颈外静脉
exteral jugular vein

颈横神经
transverse nerve of neck

颈前静脉
jugular venous vein

锁骨上神经
supraclavicular nerve

枕小神经
lesser occipital nerve

枕大神经
greater occipital nerve

耳大神经
greater auricular nerve

副神经
accessory nerve

肩胛舌骨肌下腹
inferior belly of omohyoid

臂丛
brachial plexus

图 2-19　枕三角的内容
structure of occipital triangle

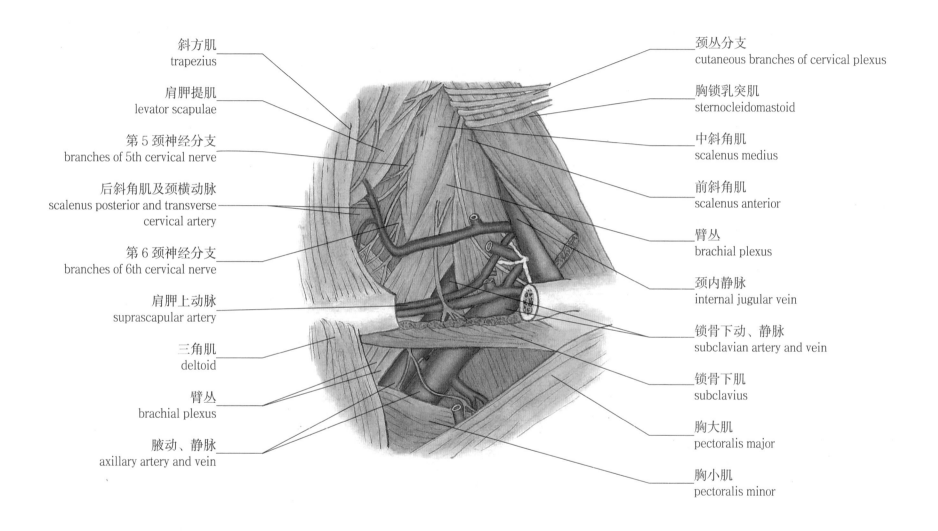

斜方肌
trapezius

肩胛提肌
levator scapulae

第 5 颈神经分支
branches of 5th cervical nerve

后斜角肌及颈横动脉
scalenus posterior and transverse
cervical artery

第 6 颈神经分支
branches of 6th cervical nerve

肩胛上动脉
suprascapular artery

三角肌
deltoid

臂丛
brachial plexus

腋动、静脉
axillary artery and vein

颈丛分支
cutaneous branches of cervical plexus

胸锁乳突肌
sternocleidomastoid

中斜角肌
scalenus medius

前斜角肌
scalenus anterior

臂丛
brachial plexus

颈内静脉
internal jugular vein

锁骨下动、静脉
subclavian artery and vein

锁骨下肌
subclavius

胸大肌
pectoralis major

胸小肌
pectoralis minor

图 2-20　肩胛舌骨肌锁骨三角内容
Omohyoid and structure of supraclavicular triangle

颏下淋巴结
submental lymph node

下颌下淋巴结
submandibular lymph node

舌骨
hyoid bone

甲状腺淋巴结
thyroid lymph node

喉前淋巴结
prelaryngeal lymph node

气管前淋巴结
pretracheal lymph node

气管旁淋巴结
paratracheal lymph node

颈前淋巴结
anterior cervical lymph node

颈内静脉肩胛舌骨
juguloomohyoid lymph node

枕淋巴结
occipital lymph node

乳突淋巴结
mastoid lymph node

腮腺淋巴结
parotid lymph node

颈外侧上深淋巴结
superior deep lateral lymph node

颈内静脉二腹肌淋巴结
jugulodigastric lymph node

颈外侧浅淋巴结
superficial lateral cervical lymph node

副神经及副神经淋巴结
accessory nerve and lymph node of accessory nerve

锁骨上淋巴结
supraclavicular lymph node

颈横动脉
transverse cervical artery

锁骨上淋巴结
subprraclavicular lymph node

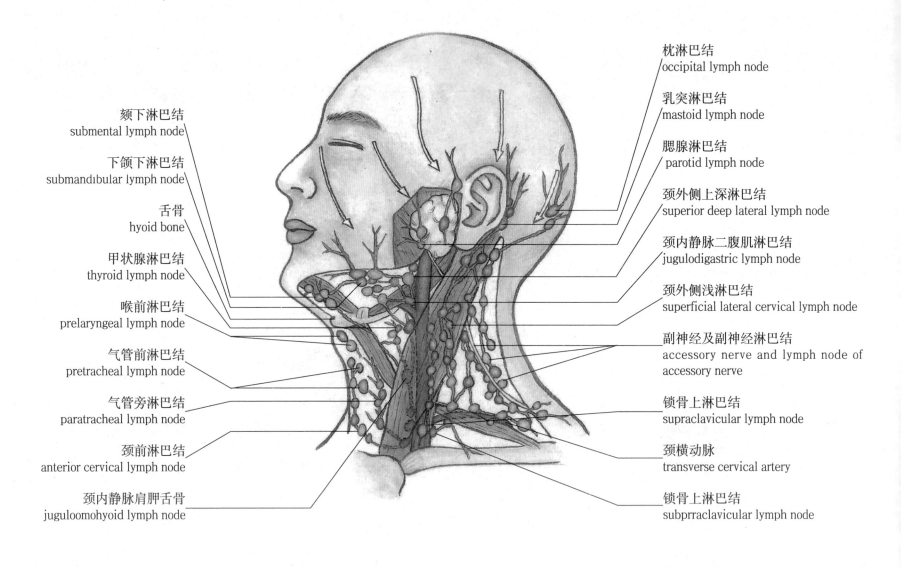

图 2-21 颈部的淋巴结
Juguloomohyoid lymph node

第三章

上肢

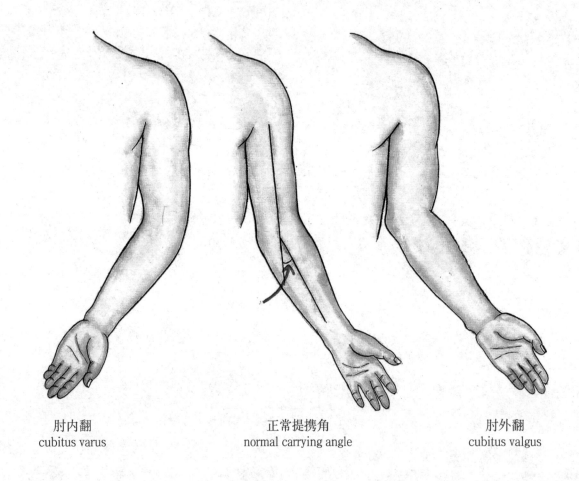

肘内翻
cubitus varus

正常提携角
normal carrying angle

肘外翻
cubitus valgus

图 3-1　提携角
Carrying angle

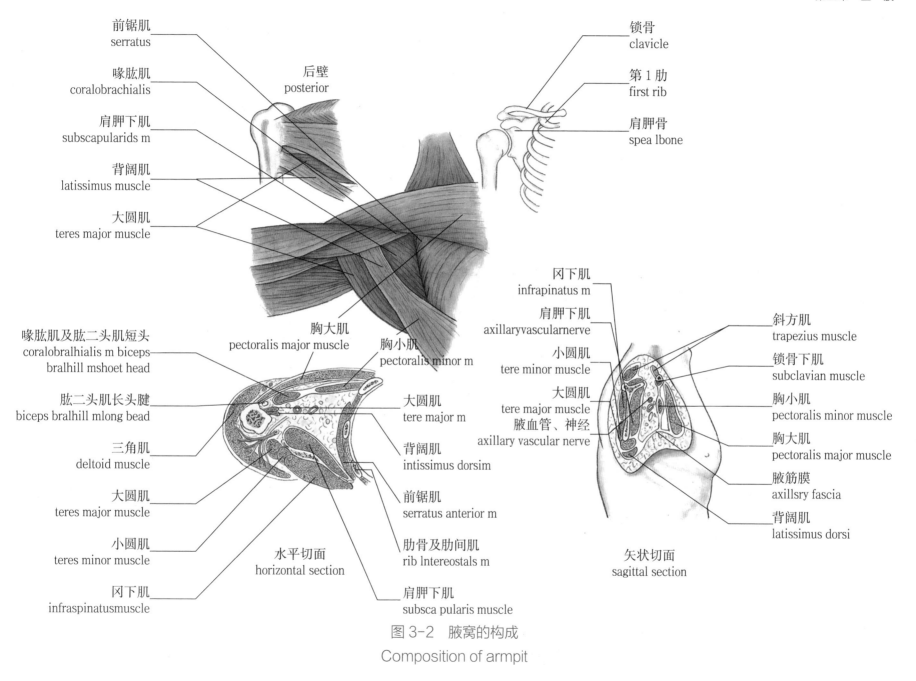

前锯肌
serratus

喙肱肌
coralobrachialis

肩胛下肌
subscapularids m

背阔肌
latissimus muscle

大圆肌
teres major muscle

后壁
posterior

锁骨
clavicle

第 1 肋
first rib

肩胛骨
spea lbone

冈下肌
infrapinatus m

肩胛下肌
axillaryvascularnerve

小圆肌
tere minor muscle

大圆肌
tere major muscle

腋血管、神经
axillary vascular nerve

斜方肌
trapezius muscle

锁骨下肌
subclavian muscle

胸小肌
pectoralis minor muscle

胸大肌
pectoralis major muscle

腋筋膜
axillsry fascia

背阔肌
latissimus dorsi

喙肱肌及肱二头肌短头
coralobralhialis m biceps
bralhill mshoet head

肱二头肌长头腱
biceps bralhill mlong bead

三角肌
deltoid muscle

大圆肌
teres major muscle

小圆肌
teres minor muscle

冈下肌
infraspinatusmuscle

胸大肌
pectoralis major muscle

胸小肌
pectoralis minor m

大圆肌
tere major m

背阔肌
intissimus dorsim

前锯肌
serratus anterior m

肋骨及肋间肌
rib lntereostals m

肩胛下肌
subsca pularis muscle

水平切面
horizontal section

矢状切面
sagittal section

图 3-2　腋窝的构成
Composition of armpit

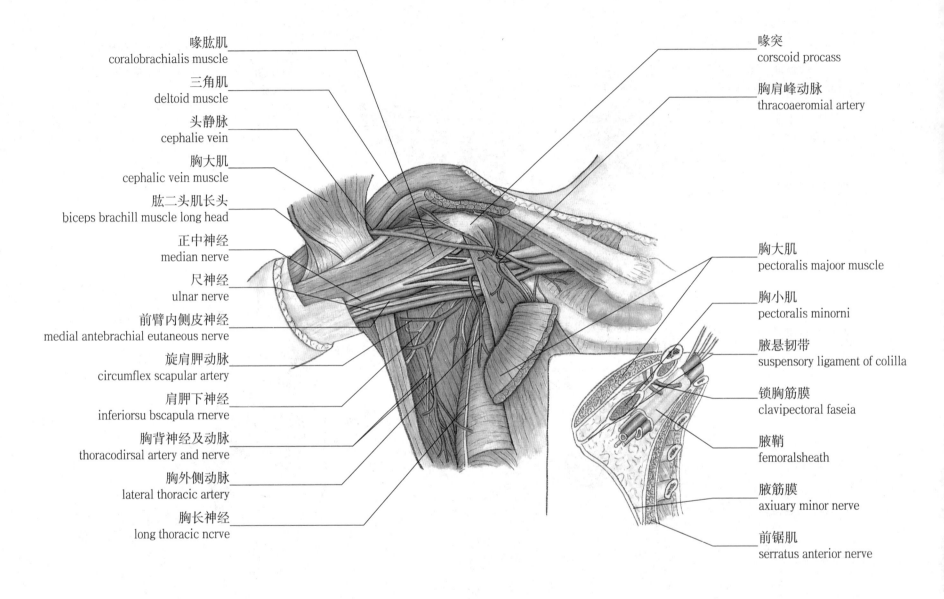

喙肱肌
coralobrachialis muscle

三角肌
deltoid muscle

头静脉
cephalie vein

胸大肌
cephalic vein muscle

肱二头肌长头
biceps brachill muscle long head

正中神经
median nerve

尺神经
ulnar nerve

前臂内侧皮神经
medial antebrachial eutaneous nerve

旋肩胛动脉
circumflex scapular artery

肩胛下神经
inferiorsu bscapula rnerve

胸背神经及动脉
thoracodirsal artery and nerve

胸外侧动脉
lateral thoracic artery

胸长神经
long thoracic ncrve

喙突
corscoid procass

胸肩峰动脉
thracoaeromial artery

胸大肌
pectoralis majoor muscle

胸小肌
pectoralis minorni

腋悬韧带
suspensory ligament of colilla

锁胸筋膜
clavipectoral faseia

腋鞘
femoralsheath

腋筋膜
axiuary minor nerve

前锯肌
serratus anterior nerve

图 3-3　腋窝前壁和内容
Anterior axillary wall and content

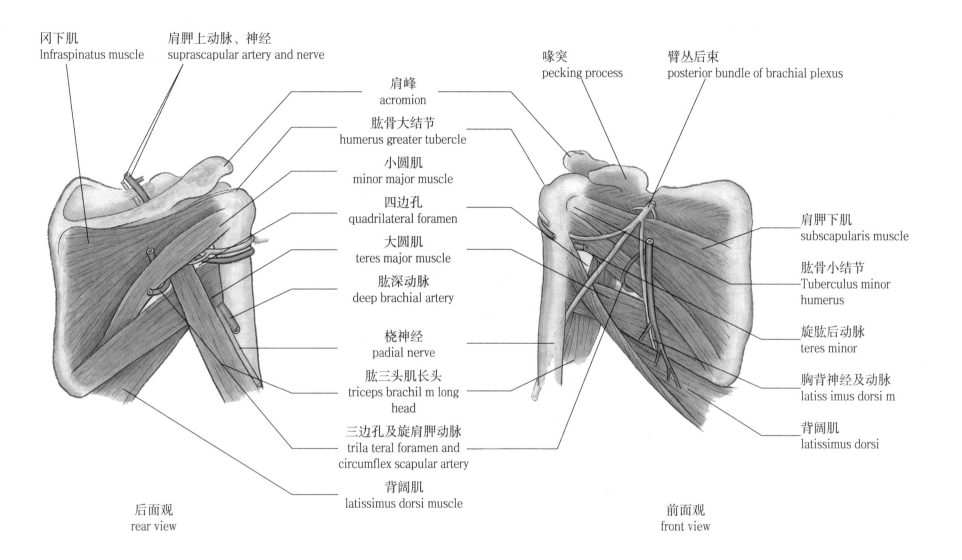

冈下肌
lnfraspinatus muscle

肩胛上动脉、神经
suprascapular artery and nerve

肩峰
acromion

肱骨大结节
humerus greater tubercle

小圆肌
minor major muscle

四边孔
quadrilateral foramen

大圆肌
teres major muscle

肱深动脉
deep brachial artery

桡神经
padial nerve

肱三头肌长头
triceps brachil m long head

三边孔及旋肩胛动脉
trila teral foramen and circumflex scapular artery

背阔肌
latissimus dorsi muscle

喙突
pecking process

臂丛后束
posterior bundle of brachial plexus

肩胛下肌
subscapularis muscle

肱骨小结节
Tuberculus minor humerus

旋肱后动脉
teres minor

胸背神经及动脉
latiss imus dorsi m

背阔肌
latissimus dorsi

后面观
rear view

前面观
front view

图 3-4　三边孔、四边孔及通过的结构
Structure through of trilateral foramen、quadrilateral foramen

肩胛背神经
dorsal scapular nerve

肩胛上神经
supra scapular nerve

肩胛上动脉
suprascapular artery

三角肌
deltoid muscle

肌皮神经
musculocutaneous nerve

旋肱前动脉
anterior circumflexbrac hialartery

腋神经
axillary nerve

正中神经
median nerve

腋动脉
axillary artery

尺神经
ulnar nerve

胸背神经及动、静脉
thoracodorsal nerve,artery and vein

胸外侧动脉
lateral thoracic artery

副神经
accessory nerve

膈神经
phrenic nerve

迷走神经
vagus nerve

颈总动脉
common carotid artery

锁骨下动脉
subclavian artery

腋动脉
axillary artery

胸肩峰动脉
thoracoacromial artery

胸上动脉
superior thoracic artery

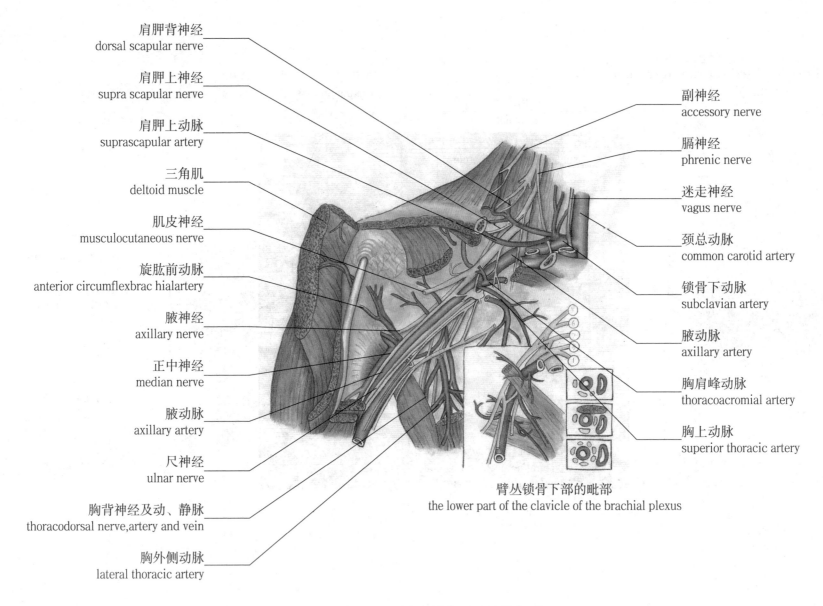

臂丛锁骨下部的毗部
the lower part of the clavicle of the brachial plexus

图 3-5　腋窝的内容及臂丛组成
Axillary content and brachial plexus composition

尖淋巴结
apical lymph nodes

外侧淋巴结
lateral lymph nodes

肩胛下淋巴结
lateral lymph nodes

中央淋巴结
central lymph node

胸肌淋巴结
pectoral lymph nodes

锁骨上淋巴结
supraclavicular lymph node

胸骨旁淋巴结
parasternal lymph nodes

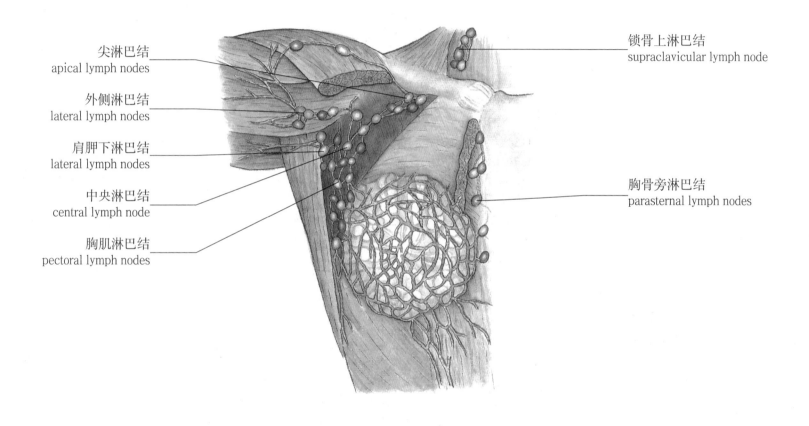

图 3-6 腋窝淋巴结
Axillary lymph node

肩胛上动脉及神经
superior scapular artery and nerve

冈上肌
supraspinatus muscle

冈下肌
infraspinatus muscle

小圆肌
teres minor

大圆肌
teres major

旋肱前动脉
anterior eiramflex humeral artery

腋动脉
axillary artery

腋神经
axillary nerve

肱骨外科颈
surgical neek of hunerus

小圆肌
teres minor

腋神经后支
potrerior branch of axillary nerve

旋肱后动脉
porterior circumflex
humeral artery

臂外侧上皮神经
superior lateral brachial
culaneous nerve

冈下肌
infrasinatus muscle

三角肌
deltoid muscle

腋神经
axillary never

四边孔
quadrilateral foramen

三边孔及旋肩胛动脉
trilateral foramen circumflex scapular
artery

肱三头肌外侧头
lateral head of triceps brachii

肱三头肌长头
long head of triceps brachii

三角肌
detoid muscle

腋神经前支
anterior branch
of axilluary never

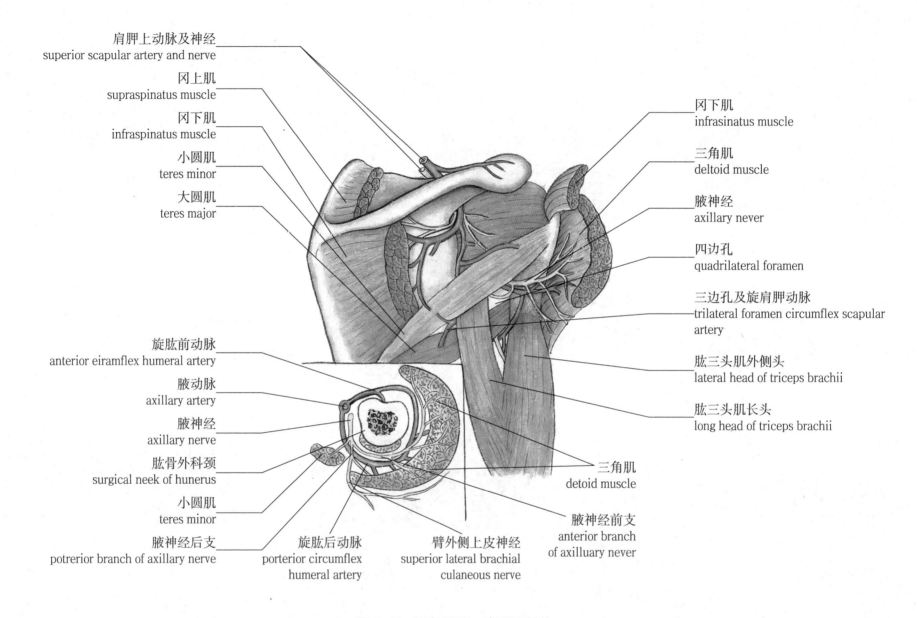

图 3-7　三角肌区、肩胛区结构
Deltoid region、scapular structure

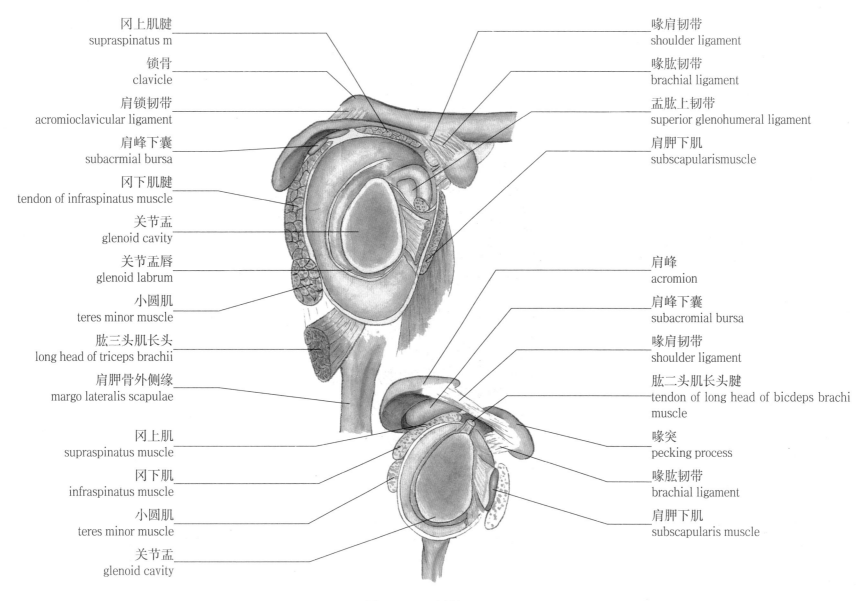

冈上肌腱
supraspinatus m

锁骨
clavicle

肩锁韧带
acromioclavicular ligament

肩峰下囊
subacrmial bursa

冈下肌腱
tendon of infraspinatus muscle

关节盂
glenoid cavity

关节盂唇
glenoid labrum

小圆肌
teres minor muscle

肱三头肌长头
long head of triceps brachii

肩胛骨外侧缘
margo lateralis scapulae

冈上肌
supraspinatus muscle

冈下肌
infraspinatus muscle

小圆肌
teres minor muscle

关节盂
glenoid cavity

喙肩韧带
shoulder ligament

喙肱韧带
brachial ligament

盂肱上韧带
superior glenohumeral ligament

肩胛下肌
subscapularismuscle

肩峰
acromion

肩峰下囊
subacromial bursa

喙肩韧带
shoulder ligament

肱二头肌长头腱
tendon of long head of bicdeps brachi muscle

喙突
pecking process

喙肱韧带
brachial ligament

肩胛下肌
subscapularis muscle

图 3-8　肌腱袖
Tendon sleeve

肩胛上动脉
superior scapular artery

肩胛背动脉
dorsal scapular artery

肩峰支
acromial branch

旋肩胛动脉
circumflex scapular artery

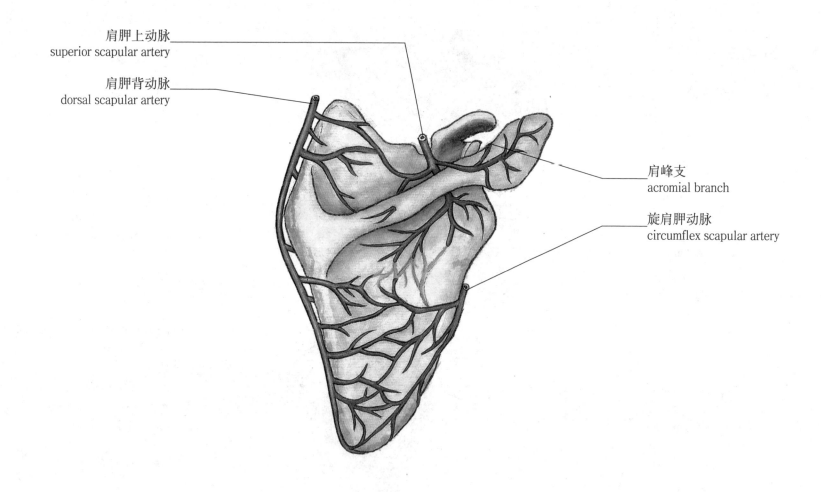

图 3-9　肩胛（周）动脉网
Circumflex scapular artery

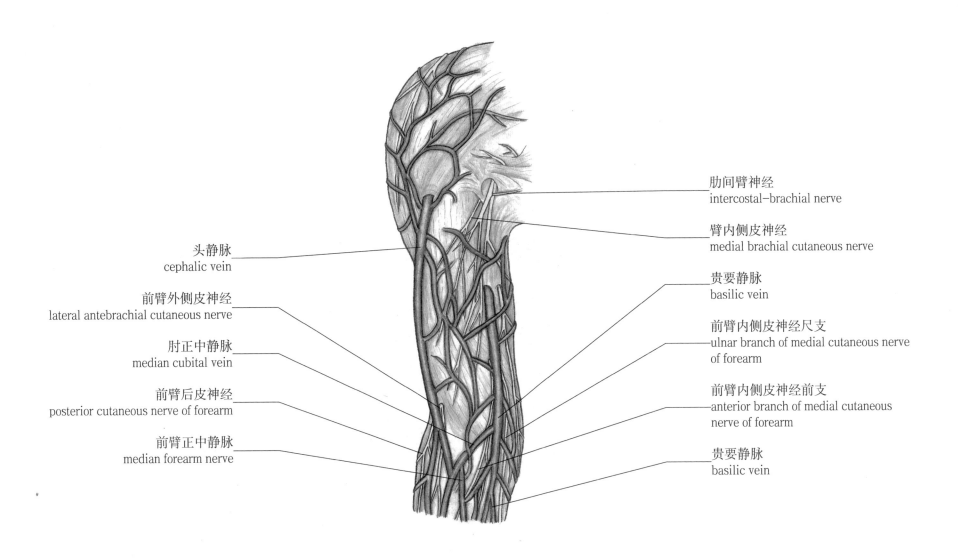

肋间臂神经
intercostal-brachial nerve

臂内侧皮神经
medial brachial cutaneous nerve

头静脉
cephalic vein

贵要静脉
basilic vein

前臂外侧皮神经
lateral antebrachial cutaneous nerve

前臂内侧皮神经尺支
ulnar branch of medial cutaneous nerve of forearm

肘正中静脉
median cubital vein

前臂后皮神经
posterior cutaneous nerve of forearm

前臂内侧皮神经前支
anterior branch of medial cutaneous nerve of forearm

前臂正中静脉
median forearm nerve

贵要静脉
basilic vein

图 3-10　臂前区浅层结构
Shallow structure of forearm region

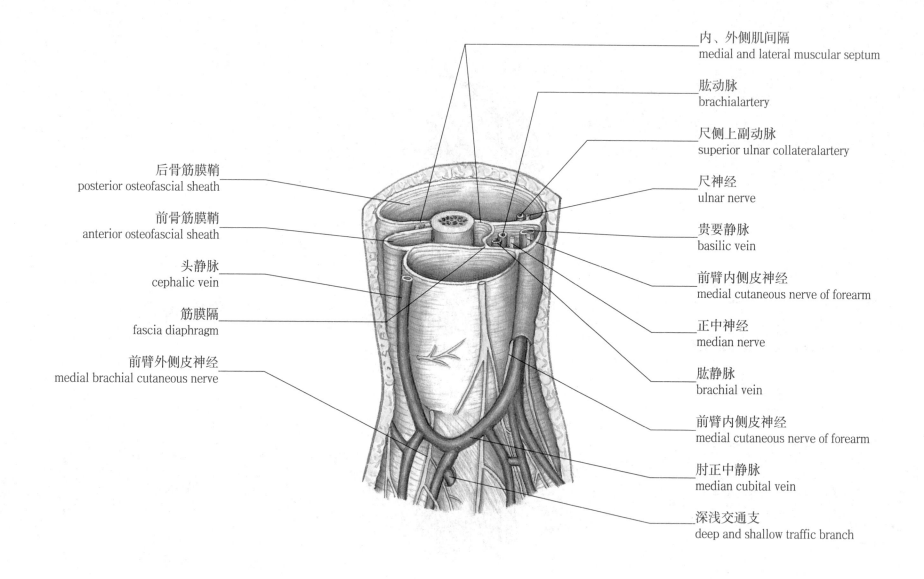

内、外侧肌间隔
medial and lateral muscular septum

肱动脉
brachialartery

尺侧上副动脉
superior ulnar collateralartery

尺神经
ulnar nerve

贵要静脉
basilic vein

前臂内侧皮神经
medial cutaneous nerve of forearm

正中神经
median nerve

肱静脉
brachial vein

前臂内侧皮神经
medial cutaneous nerve of forearm

肘正中静脉
median cubital vein

深浅交通支
deep and shallow traffic branch

后骨筋膜鞘
posterior osteofascial sheath

前骨筋膜鞘
anterior osteofascial sheath

头静脉
cephalic vein

筋膜隔
fascia diaphragm

前臂外侧皮神经
medial brachial cutaneous nerve

图 3-11 臂部骨筋膜鞘
Osteofascial sheath of arm

三角肌
deltoid muscle

喙肱肌
coracobrachialis muscle

肌皮神经
musculocutaneous nerve

肱二头肌长头
biceps brachii long head

肱二头肌短头
biceps brachii short head

肱肌
brachial muscle

肱二头肌
biceos brachii m

前臂外侧皮神经
lateral anterbachial cutaneous n

桡神经深支
deep branch of radial nerve

旋后肌
supinator muscle

正中神经
median nerve

桡动脉
radial artery

桡神经浅支
superficial branch of radial nerve

腋动脉
axillary artery

尺神经
ulnar nerve

肋间臂神经
intercostal brachial nerve

前臂内侧皮神经
medial cutancous nerve of forcarm

尺侧上副动脉
superoir ulnar collateral artery

肱二头肌腱
biceps tendon

旋前圆肌肱头
pronator teresm （humeral bead）

旋前圆肌尺头
pronator teresm（ulnar head）

指浅屈肌肱尺头
caput humero–ulnare musculi flexoris digitorum superficialis

指浅屈肌桡头
flexor digtorum supperficidlis muscle （radia head）

尺神经
ulnar nerve

尺动脉
ulnar artery

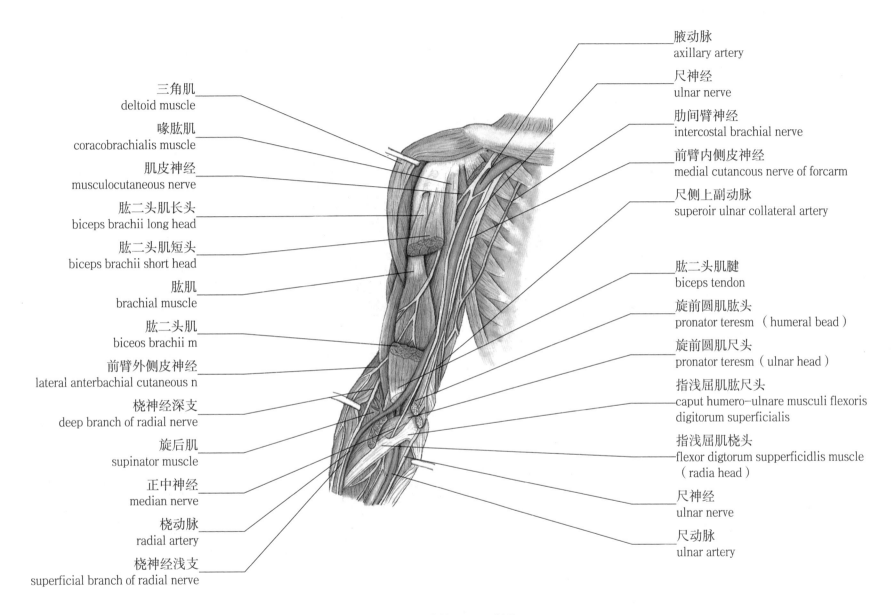

图 3-12　臂前区深层结构
Deepstr ucture of forear mregion

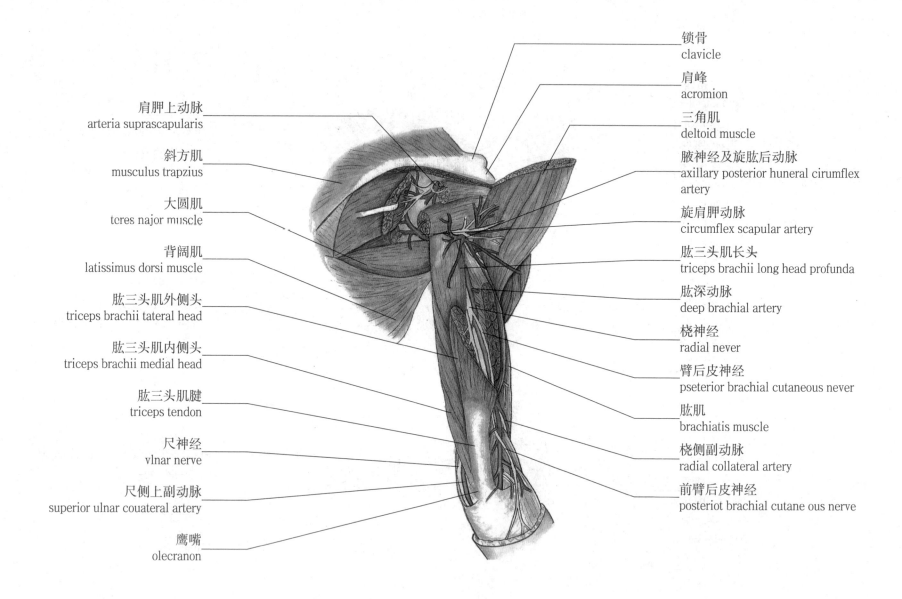

肩胛上动脉
arteria suprascapularis

斜方肌
musculus trapzius

大圆肌
tcres najor muscle

背阔肌
latissimus dorsi muscle

肱三头肌外侧头
triceps brachii tateral head

肱三头肌内侧头
triceps brachii medial head

肱三头肌腱
triceps tendon

尺神经
vlnar nerve

尺侧上副动脉
superior ulnar couateral artery

鹰嘴
olecranon

锁骨
clavicle

肩峰
acromion

三角肌
deltoid muscle

腋神经及旋肱后动脉
axillary posterior huneral cirumflex artery

旋肩胛动脉
circumflex scapular artery

肱三头肌长头
triceps brachii long head profunda

肱深动脉
deep brachial artery

桡神经
radial never

臂后皮神经
pseterior brachial cutaneous never

肱肌
brachiatis muscle

桡侧副动脉
radial collateral artery

前臂后皮神经
posteriot brachial cutane ous nerve

图 3-13　臂后区深层结构
Deep structure of posterior brachial region

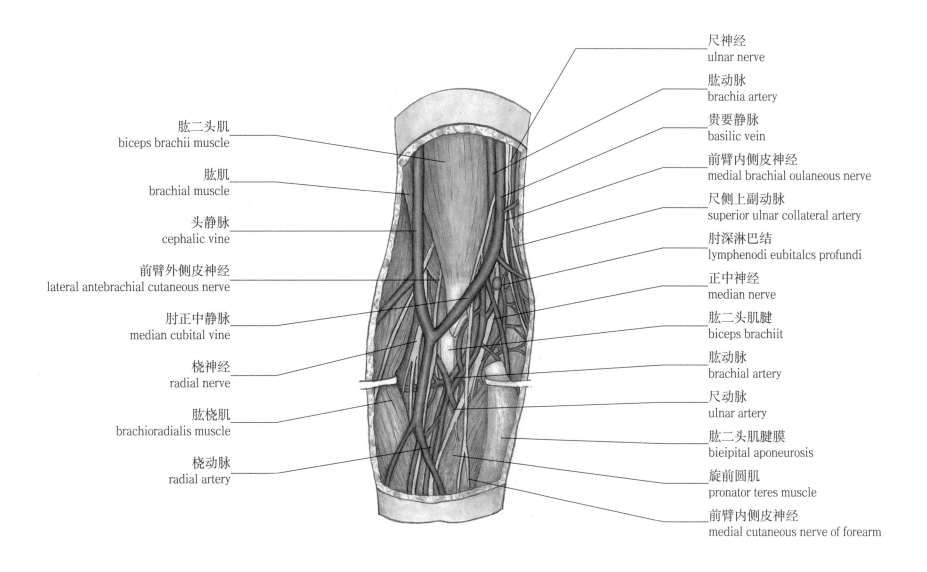

肱二头肌
biceps brachii muscle

肱肌
brachial muscle

头静脉
cephalic vine

前臂外侧皮神经
lateral antebrachial cutaneous nerve

肘正中静脉
median cubital vine

桡神经
radial nerve

肱桡肌
brachioradialis muscle

桡动脉
radial artery

尺神经
ulnar nerve

肱动脉
brachia artery

贵要静脉
basilic vein

前臂内侧皮神经
medial brachial oulaneous nerve

尺侧上副动脉
superior ulnar collateral artery

肘深淋巴结
lymphenodi eubitalcs profundi

正中神经
median nerve

肱二头肌腱
biceps brachiit

肱动脉
brachial artery

尺动脉
ulnar artery

肱二头肌腱膜
bieipital aponeurosis

旋前圆肌
pronator teres muscle

前臂内侧皮神经
medial cutaneous nerve of forearm

图 3-14　肘前区及前臂前区的浅层结构
Deep stercuture of posterior brachial region

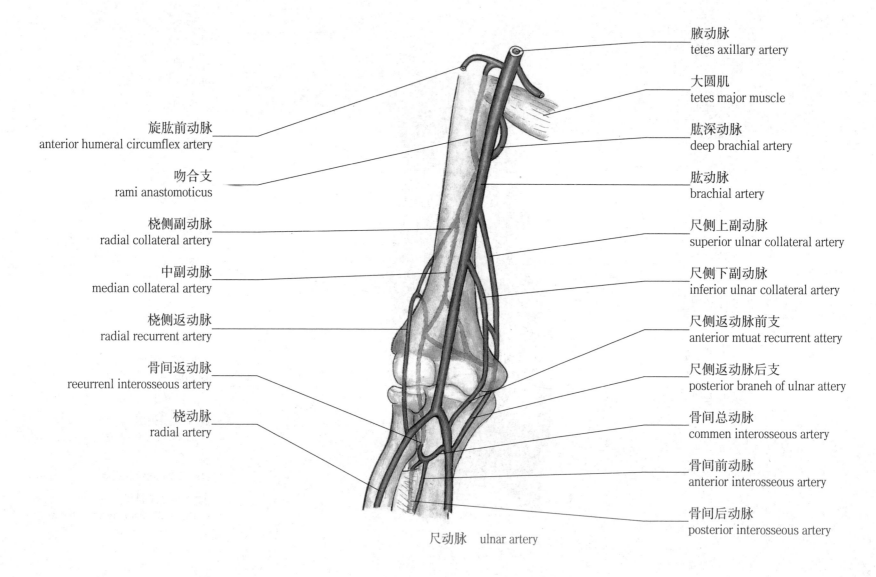

腋动脉
tetes axillary artery

大圆肌
tetes major muscle

肱深动脉
deep brachial artery

肱动脉
brachial artery

尺侧上副动脉
superior ulnar collateral artery

尺侧下副动脉
inferior ulnar collateral artery

尺侧返动脉前支
anterior mtuat recurrent attery

尺侧返动脉后支
posterior braneh of ulnar attery

骨间总动脉
commen interosseous artery

骨间前动脉
anterior interosseous artery

骨间后动脉
posterior interosseous artery

旋肱前动脉
anterior humeral circumflex artery

吻合支
rami anastomoticus

桡侧副动脉
radial collateral artery

中副动脉
median collateral artery

桡侧返动脉
radial recurrent artery

骨间返动脉
reeurrenl interosseous artery

桡动脉
radial artery

尺动脉　ulnar artery

图 3-15　肘关节动脉网
Aretrial network of elbow joint

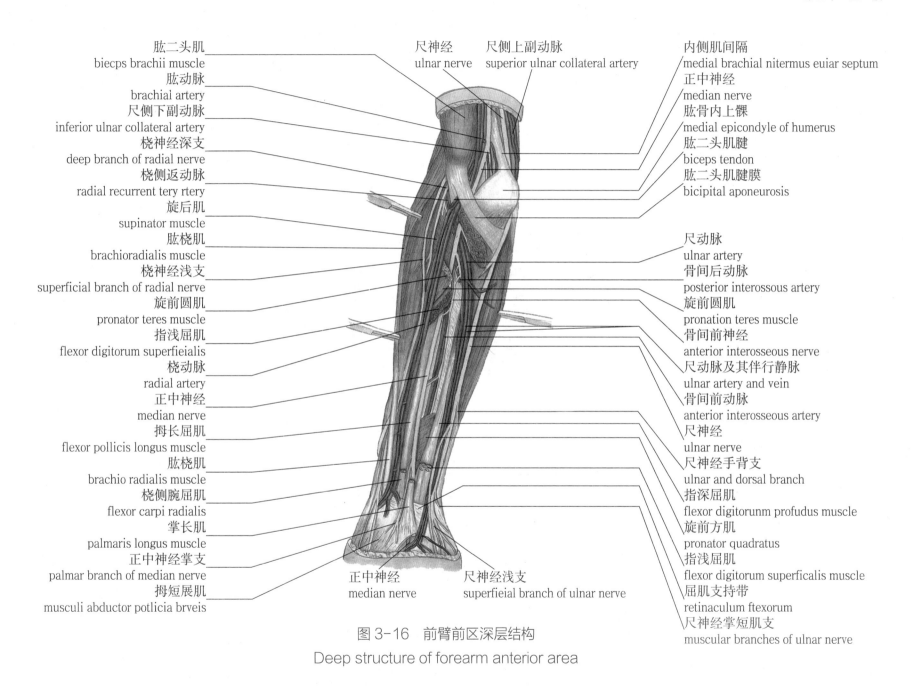

肱二头肌
biecps brachii muscle

肱动脉
brachial artery

尺侧下副动脉
inferior ulnar collateral artery

桡神经深支
deep branch of radial nerve

桡侧返动脉
radial recurrent tery rtery

旋后肌
supinator muscle

肱桡肌
brachioradialis muscle

桡神经浅支
superficial branch of radial nerve

旋前圆肌
pronator teres muscle

指浅屈肌
flexor digitorum superfieialis

桡动脉
radial artery

正中神经
median nerve

拇长屈肌
flexor pollicis longus muscle

肱桡肌
brachio radialis muscle

桡侧腕屈肌
flexor carpi radialis

掌长肌
palmaris longus muscle

正中神经掌支
palmar branch of median nerve

拇短展肌
musculi abductor potlicia brveis

尺神经
ulnar nerve

尺侧上副动脉
superior ulnar collateral artery

内侧肌间隔
medial brachial nitermus euiar septum

正中神经
median nerve

肱骨内上髁
medial epicondyle of humerus

肱二头肌腱
biceps tendon

肱二头肌腱膜
bicipital aponeurosis

尺动脉
ulnar artery

骨间后动脉
posterior interossous artery

旋前圆肌
pronation teres muscle

骨间前神经
anterior interosseous nerve

尺动脉及其伴行静脉
ulnar artery and vein

骨间前动脉
anterior interosseous artery

尺神经
ulnar nerve

尺神经手背支
ulnar and dorsal branch

指深屈肌
flexor digitorunm profudus muscle

旋前方肌
pronator quadratus

指浅屈肌
flexor digitorum superficalis muscle

屈肌支持带
retinaculum ftexorum

尺神经掌短肌支
muscular branches of ulnar nerve

正中神经
median nerve

尺神经浅支
superfieial branch of ulnar nerve

图 3-16 前臂前区深层结构
Deep structure of forearm anterior area

桡侧腕长伸肌
extensor carpi radialis longus mussole

旋后肌
supinator muscle

桡侧腕短伸肌
extensor carpi radialis brevis muscle

骨间后动脉
posterior interosseous artery

指伸肌
museulus extensor digitorum

骨间后神经
posterior interosseous nerve

拇长伸肌
extensor pouieis longus muscle

尺侧腕伸肌
extensor carpi ulnarist

小指伸肌
extensor digti minimi

伸肌支持带
extensor retinaculum

肘肌
anecneus

桡神经
radial nerve

桡神经深支
radial deep branch

桡神经浅支
radial supeerfieial

旋后肌
supinator muscle

旋前圆肌
tendon of abduetor pallicis brevis muscle

拇长展肌
tendon of extensor pallieis brevis muscle

拇短伸肌
tendon of extensor pallieis brevis muscle

解剖学"鼻烟窝"
anatomical sruffbox

桡动脉
radial artery

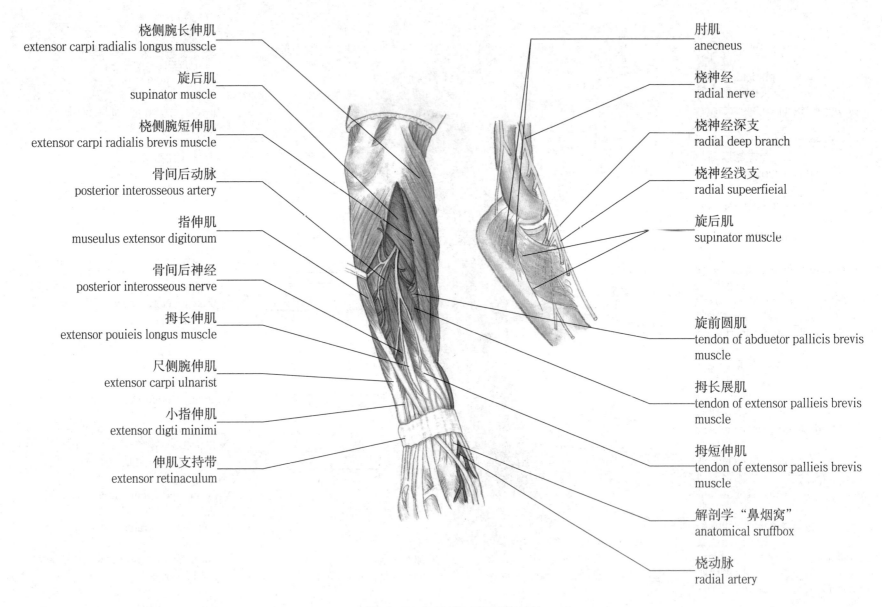

图 3-17　前臂后区深层结构
Deep structure of posterior forearm

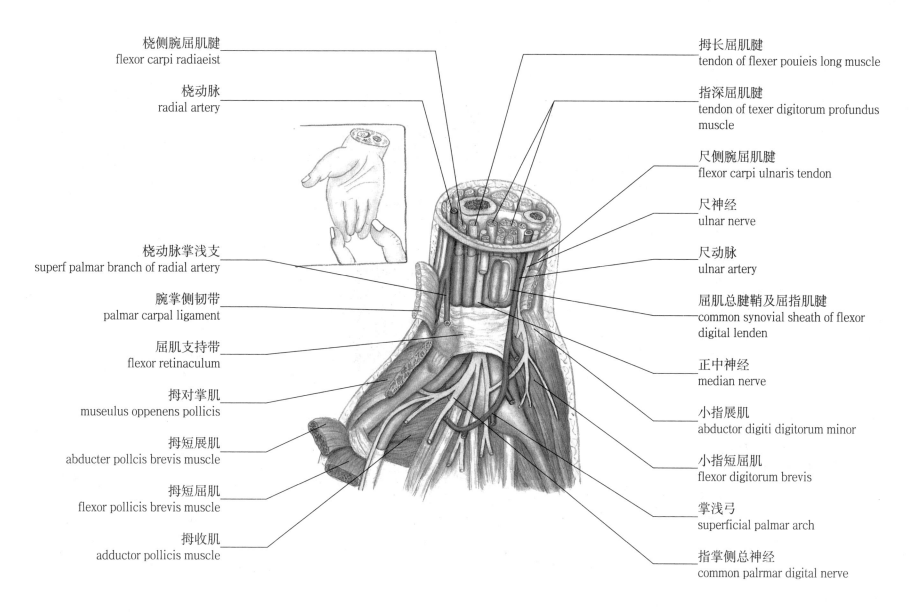

桡侧腕屈肌腱
flexor carpi radiaeist

桡动脉
radial artery

桡动脉掌浅支
superf palmar branch of radial artery

腕掌侧韧带
palmar carpal ligament

屈肌支持带
flexor retinaculum

拇对掌肌
museulus oppenens pollicis

拇短展肌
abducter pollcis brevis muscle

拇短屈肌
flexor pollicis brevis muscle

拇收肌
adductor pollicis muscle

拇长屈肌腱
tendon of flexer pouieis long muscle

指深屈肌腱
tendon of texer digitorum profundus muscle

尺侧腕屈肌腱
flexor carpi ulnaris tendon

尺神经
ulnar nerve

尺动脉
ulnar artery

屈肌总腱鞘及屈指肌腱
common synovial sheath of flexor digital lenden

正中神经
median nerve

小指展肌
abductor digiti digitorum minor

小指短屈肌
flexor digitorum brevis

掌浅弓
superficial palmar arch

指掌侧总神经
common palrmar digital nerve

图 3-18　腕前区深层结构
Deep structure of anterior carpal region

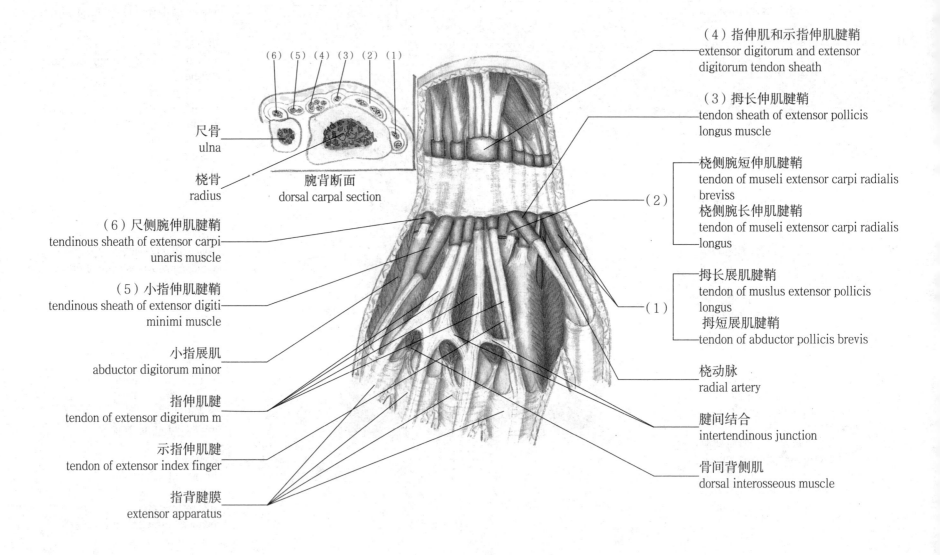

（4）指伸肌和示指伸肌腱鞘
extensor digitorum and extensor digitorum tendon sheath

（3）拇长伸肌腱鞘
tendon sheath of extensor pollicis longus muscle

桡侧腕短伸肌腱鞘
tendon of museli extensor carpi radialis breviss

桡侧腕长伸肌腱鞘
tendon of museli extensor carpi radialis longus

（2）

拇长展肌腱鞘
tendon of muslus extensor pollicis longus

拇短展肌腱鞘
tendon of abductor pollicis brevis

（1）

桡动脉
radial artery

腱间结合
intertendinous junction

骨间背侧肌
dorsal interosseous muscle

(6)(5)(4)(3)(2)(1)

尺骨
ulna

桡骨
radius

腕背断面
dorsal carpal section

（6）尺侧腕伸肌腱鞘
tendinous sheath of extensor carpi unaris muscle

（5）小指伸肌腱鞘
tendinous sheath of extensor digiti minimi muscle

小指展肌
abductor digitorum minor

指伸肌腱
tendon of extensor digiterum m

示指伸肌腱
tendon of extensor index finger

指背腱膜
extensor apparatus

图 3-19　腕后区及手背深层结构
Deep structure of posterior carpal region dorsum of hand

指浅屈肌
tenden of flexor digitorun
superficiatis musc

饶侧腕屈肌
flexer rarpi radialis

桡动脉
radial artery

桡神经浅支
superficial branch of radial nerve

掌腱膜
palmar aponeurosis

指掌侧总动脉
arterie digitales palmares communes

指掌侧固有动脉、神经
plmar digital artery and nerve

尺动脉
ulnar artery

尺神经
ulnar nerve

掌长肌腱
palmaris longus

屈肌支持带
retinacutum

掌短肌
palmaris brevis muscle

指蹼间隙
finger web space

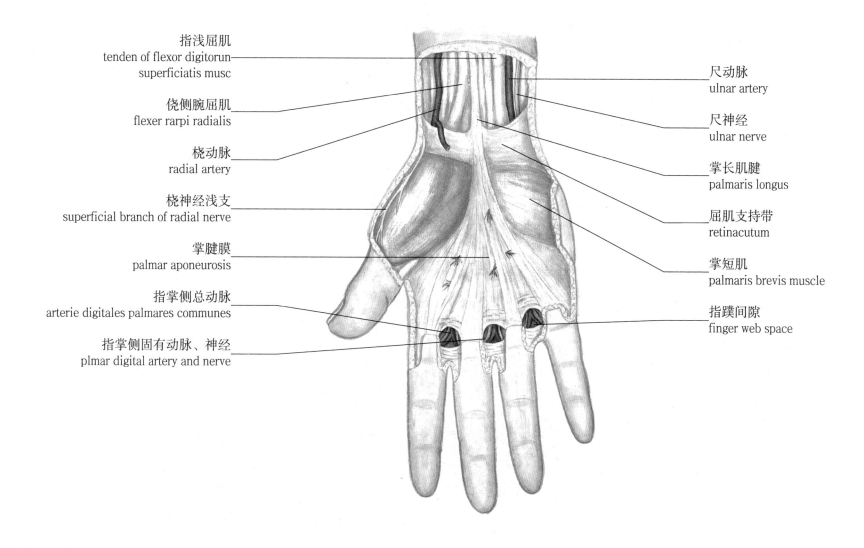

图 3-20　掌腱膜
Palmar aponeurosis

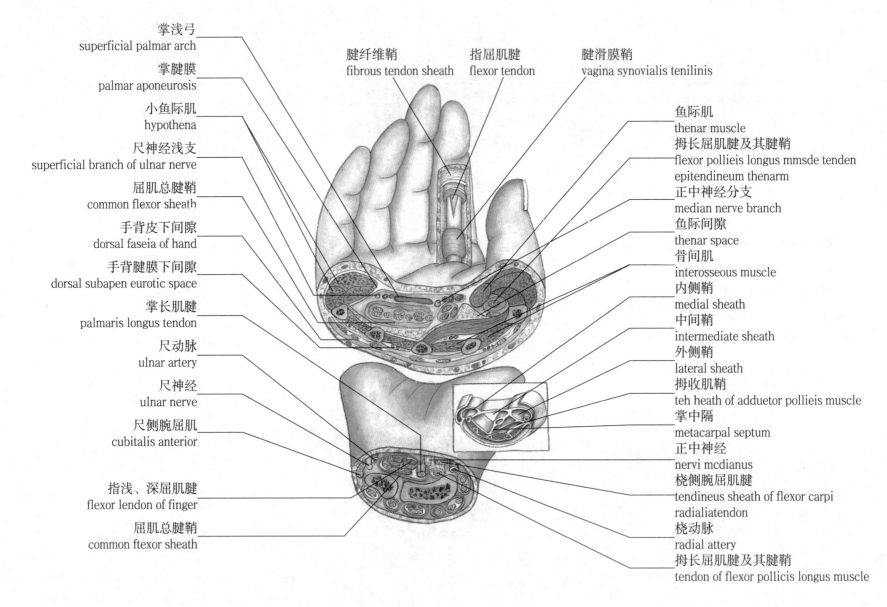

掌浅弓
superficial palmar arch

掌腱膜
palmar aponeurosis

小鱼际肌
hypothena

尺神经浅支
superficial branch of ulnar nerve

屈肌总腱鞘
common flexor sheath

手背皮下间隙
dorsal faseia of hand

手背腱膜下间隙
dorsal subapen eurotic space

掌长肌腱
palmaris longus tendon

尺动脉
ulnar artery

尺神经
ulnar nerve

尺侧腕屈肌
cubitalis anterior

指浅、深屈肌腱
flexor lendon of finger

屈肌总腱鞘
common ftexor sheath

腱纤维鞘
fibrous tendon sheath

指屈肌腱
flexor tendon

腱滑膜鞘
vagina synovialis tenilinis

鱼际肌
thenar muscle

拇长屈肌腱及其腱鞘
flexor pollieis longus mmsde tenden epitendineum thenarm

正中神经分支
median nerve branch

鱼际间隙
thenar space

骨间肌
interosseous muscle

内侧鞘
medial sheath

中间鞘
intermediate sheath

外侧鞘
lateral sheath

拇收肌鞘
teh heath of adduetor pollieis muscle

掌中隔
metacarpal septum

正中神经
nervi mcdianus

桡侧腕屈肌腱
tendineus sheath of flexor carpi radialiatendon

桡动脉
radial attery

拇长屈肌腱及其腱鞘
tendon of flexor pollicis longus muscle

图 3-21 手部骨筋膜鞘及内容
Hand osteofascial sheath and its contents

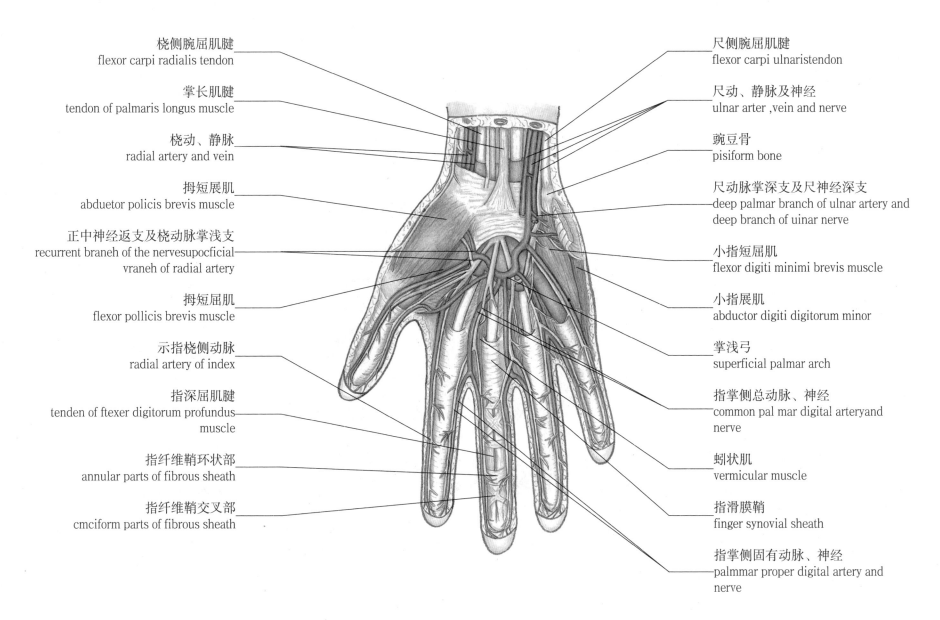

桡侧腕屈肌腱
flexor carpi radialis tendon

掌长肌腱
tendon of palmaris longus muscle

桡动、静脉
radial artery and vein

拇短展肌
abduetor policis brevis muscle

正中神经返支及桡动脉掌浅支
recurrent braneh of the nervesupocficial
vraneh of radial artery

拇短屈肌
flexor pollicis brevis muscle

示指桡侧动脉
radial artery of index

指深屈肌腱
tenden of ftexer digitorum profundus
muscle

指纤维鞘环状部
annular parts of fibrous sheath

指纤维鞘交叉部
cmciform parts of fibrous sheath

尺侧腕屈肌腱
flexor carpi ulnaristendon

尺动、静脉及神经
ulnar arter ,vein and nerve

豌豆骨
pisiform bone

尺动脉掌深支及尺神经深支
deep palmar branch of ulnar artery and
deep branch of uinar nerve

小指短屈肌
flexor digiti minimi brevis muscle

小指展肌
abductor digiti digitorum minor

掌浅弓
superficial palmar arch

指掌侧总动脉、神经
common pal mar digital arteryand
nerve

蚓状肌
vermicular muscle

指滑膜鞘
finger synovial sheath

指掌侧固有动脉、神经
palmmar proper digital artery and
nerve

图 3-22 手肌、掌浅弓和正中神经及其分支
hand muscle,superficial palmar arch,median nerve and their branches

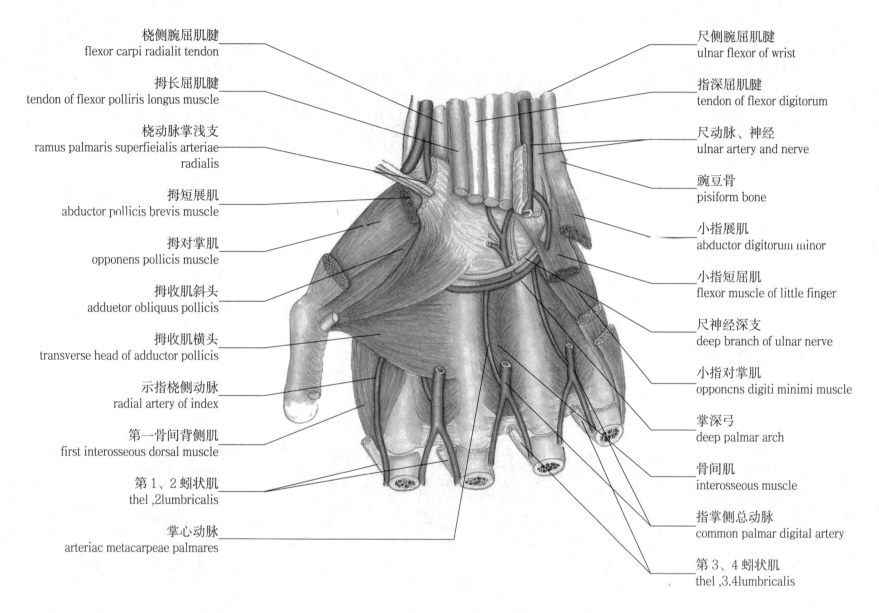

桡侧腕屈肌腱
flexor carpi radialit tendon

拇长屈肌腱
tendon of flexor polliris longus muscle

桡动脉掌浅支
ramus palmaris superfieialis arteriae radialis

拇短展肌
abductor pollicis brevis muscle

拇对掌肌
opponens pollicis muscle

拇收肌斜头
adduetor obliquus pollicis

拇收肌横头
transverse head of adductor pollicis

示指桡侧动脉
radial artery of index

第一骨间背侧肌
first interosseous dorsal muscle

第1、2蚓状肌
the1 ,2lumbricalis

掌心动脉
arteriac metacarpeae palmares

尺侧腕屈肌腱
ulnar flexor of wrist

指深屈肌腱
tendon of flexor digitorum

尺动脉、神经
ulnar artery and nerve

豌豆骨
pisiform bone

小指展肌
abductor digitorum minor

小指短屈肌
flexor muscle of little finger

尺神经深支
deep branch of ulnar nerve

小指对掌肌
opponcns digiti minimi muscle

掌深弓
deep palmar arch

骨间肌
interosseous muscle

指掌侧总动脉
common palmar digital artery

第3、4蚓状肌
the1 ,3.4lumbricalis

图 3-23　掌深弓和尺中神经
Deep palmar arch and middle ulnar nerve

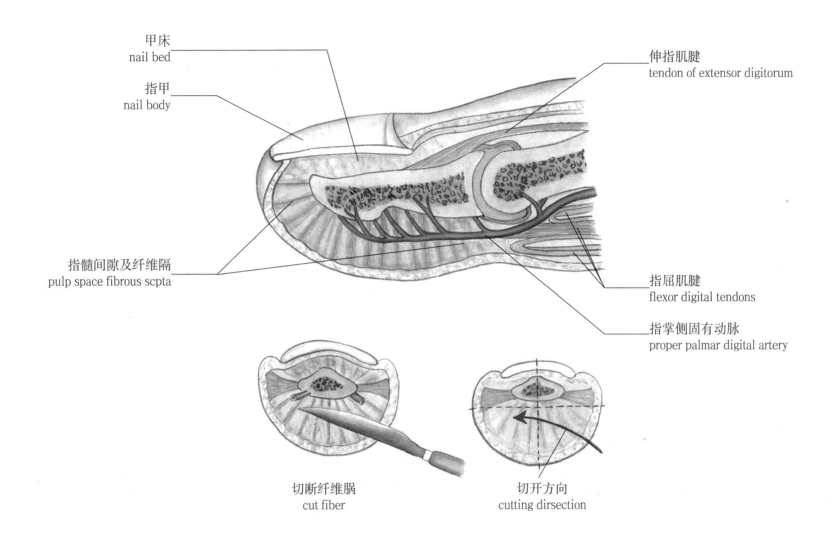

甲床
nail bed

指甲
nail body

伸指肌腱
tendon of extensor digitorum

指髓间隙及纤维隔
pulp space fibrous scpta

指屈肌腱
flexor digital tendons

指掌侧固有动脉
proper palmar digital artery

切断纤维膈
cut fiber

切开方向
cutting dirsection

图 3-24　指端结构和切开引流术
Fingrt tip structure and incision and drainage

第四章

下肢

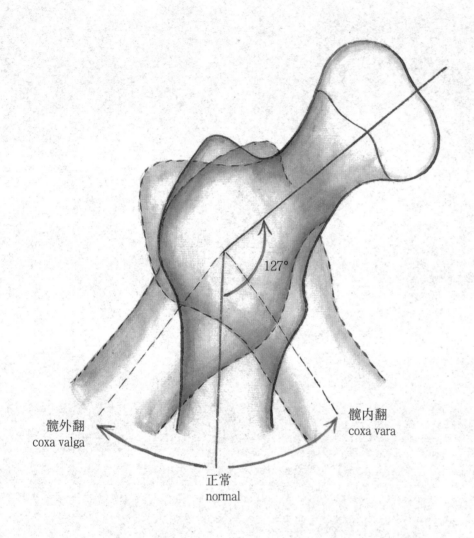

图 4-1 股骨颈干角
femoral neck shaft angle

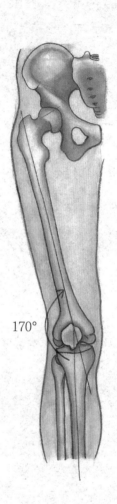

图 4-2 膝外翻角
Knee valga angle

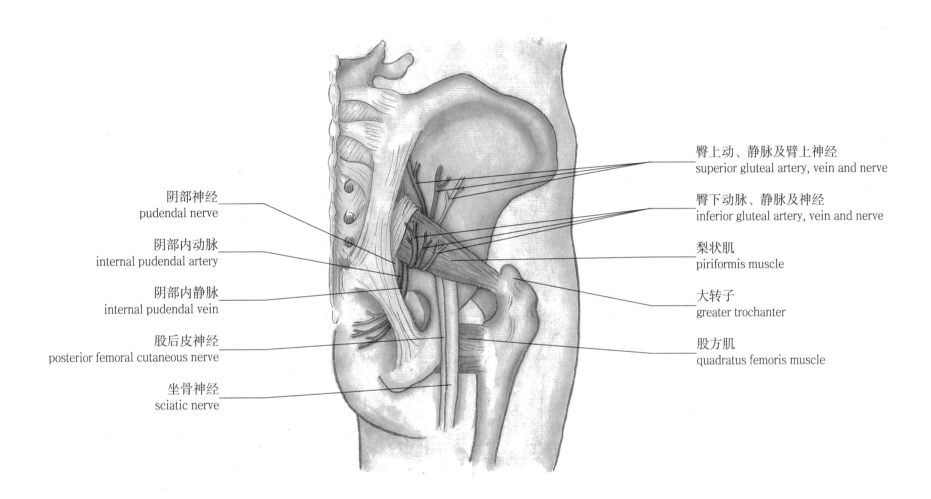

臀上动、静脉及臀上神经
superior gluteal artery, vein and nerve

臀下动脉、静脉及神经
inferior gluteal artery, vein and nerve

梨状肌
piriformis muscle

大转子
greater trochanter

股方肌
quadratus femoris muscle

阴部神经
pudendal nerve

阴部内动脉
internal pudendal artery

阴部内静脉
internal pudendal vein

股后皮神经
posterior femoral cutaneous nerve

坐骨神经
sciatic nerve

图 4-3 臀部血管神经
Hip blood vessels and nerves

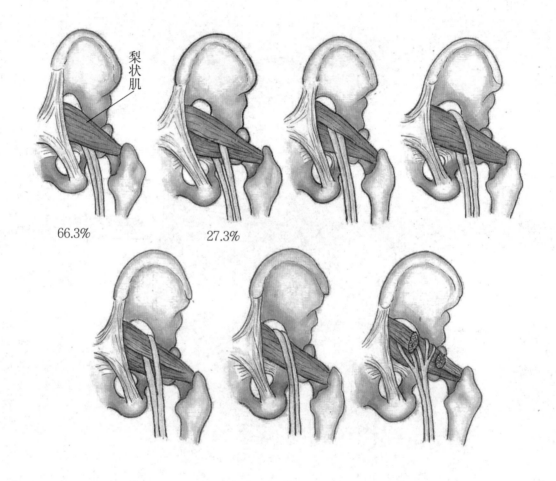

梨状肌

66.3%　　27.3%

图 4-4　坐骨神经与梨状肌关系
Relationship between sciatic nerve and piriformis muscle

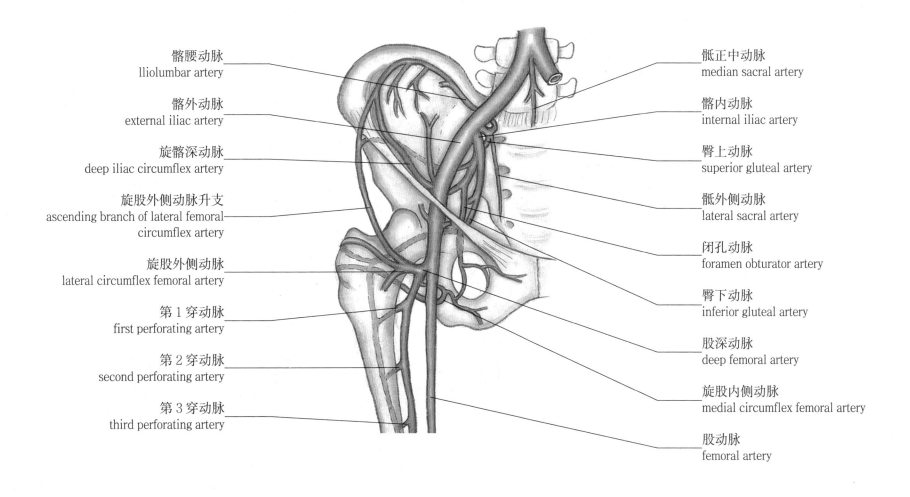

髂腰动脉
lliolumbar artery

髂外动脉
external iliac artery

旋髂深动脉
deep iliac circumflex artery

旋股外侧动脉升支
ascending branch of lateral femoral circumflex artery

旋股外侧动脉
lateral circumflex femoral artery

第 1 穿动脉
first perforating artery

第 2 穿动脉
second perforating artery

第 3 穿动脉
third perforating artery

骶正中动脉
median sacral artery

髂内动脉
internal iliac artery

臀上动脉
superior gluteal artery

骶外侧动脉
lateral sacral artery

闭孔动脉
foramen obturator artery

臀下动脉
inferior gluteal artery

股深动脉
deep femoral artery

旋股内侧动脉
medial circumflex femoral artery

股动脉
femoral artery

图 4-5 髋周围动脉网
Peri hip arterial network

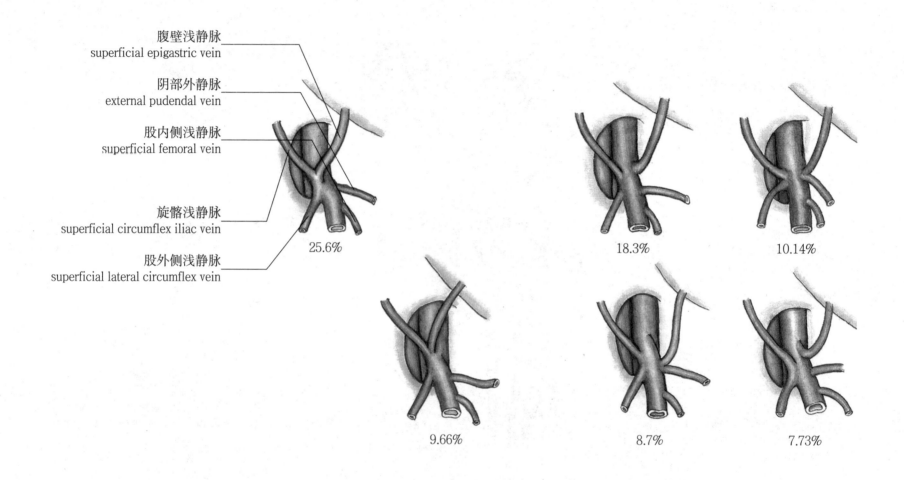

腹壁浅静脉
superficial epigastric vein

阴部外静脉
external pudendal vein

股内侧浅静脉
superficial femoral vein

旋髂浅静脉
superficial circumflex iliac vein

股外侧浅静脉
superficial lateral circumflex vein

25.6%

18.3%

10.14%

9.66%

8.7%

7.73%

图 4-6　大隐静脉上段属支的类型

The superior segment of great saphenous vein belongs to the type of branch

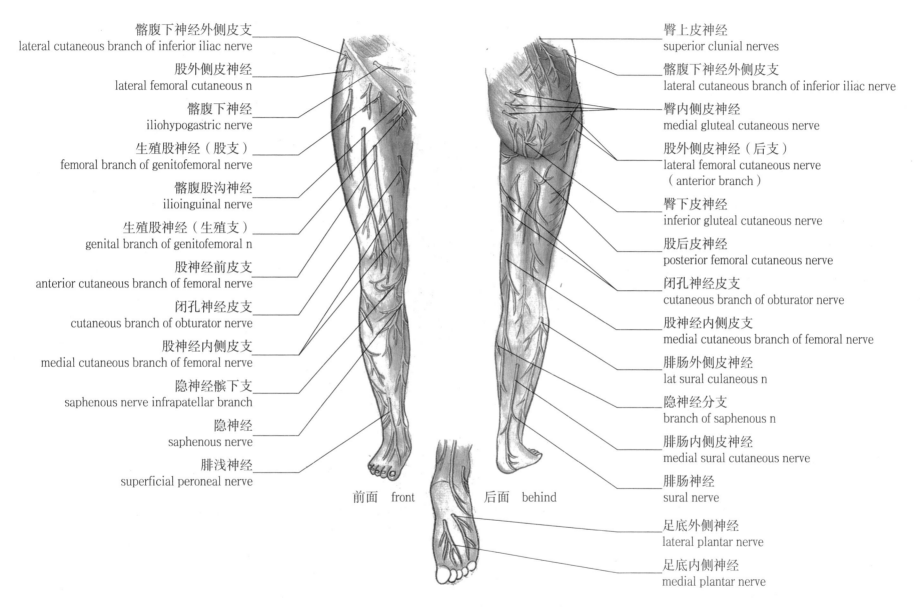

髂腹下神经外侧皮支
lateral cutaneous branch of inferior iliac nerve

股外侧皮神经
lateral femoral cutaneous n

髂腹下神经
iliohypogastric nerve

生殖股神经（股支）
femoral branch of genitofemoral nerve

髂腹股沟神经
ilioinguinal nerve

生殖股神经（生殖支）
genital branch of genitofemoral n

股神经前皮支
anterior cutaneous branch of femoral nerve

闭孔神经皮支
cutaneous branch of obturator nerve

股神经内侧皮支
medial cutaneous branch of femoral nerve

隐神经髌下支
saphenous nerve infrapatellar branch

隐神经
saphenous nerve

腓浅神经
superficial peroneal nerve

臀上皮神经
superior clunial nerves

髂腹下神经外侧皮支
lateral cutaneous branch of inferior iliac nerve

臀内侧皮神经
medial gluteal cutaneous nerve

股外侧皮神经（后支）
lateral femoral cutaneous nerve
（anterior branch）

臀下皮神经
inferior gluteal cutaneous nerve

股后皮神经
posterior femoral cutaneous nerve

闭孔神经皮支
cutaneous branch of obturator nerve

股神经内侧皮支
medial cutaneous branch of femoral nerve

腓肠外侧皮神经
lat sural culaneous n

隐神经分支
branch of saphenous n

腓肠内侧皮神经
medial sural cutaneous nerve

腓肠神经
sural nerve

足底外侧神经
lateral plantar nerve

足底内侧神经
medial plantar nerve

前面 front

后面 behind

图 4-7 下肢皮神经
Cutaneous nerve of lower extremity

髂前上棘
anterior superior iliac spine

腹股沟上外侧浅淋巴结
superficial superior lateral inguinal
lymph nodes

股静脉
femoral vein

腹股沟下外侧浅淋巴结
inferior lateral superficial inguinal
lymph nodes

髂外动、静脉及髂外淋巴结
external iliac artery, vein and external
iliac lymph node

腹股沟上内侧浅淋巴结
superior medial superficial inguinal
lymph nodes

腹股沟下内侧浅淋巴结
inferior medial superficial inguinal
lymph nodes

大隐静脉
great saphenous vein

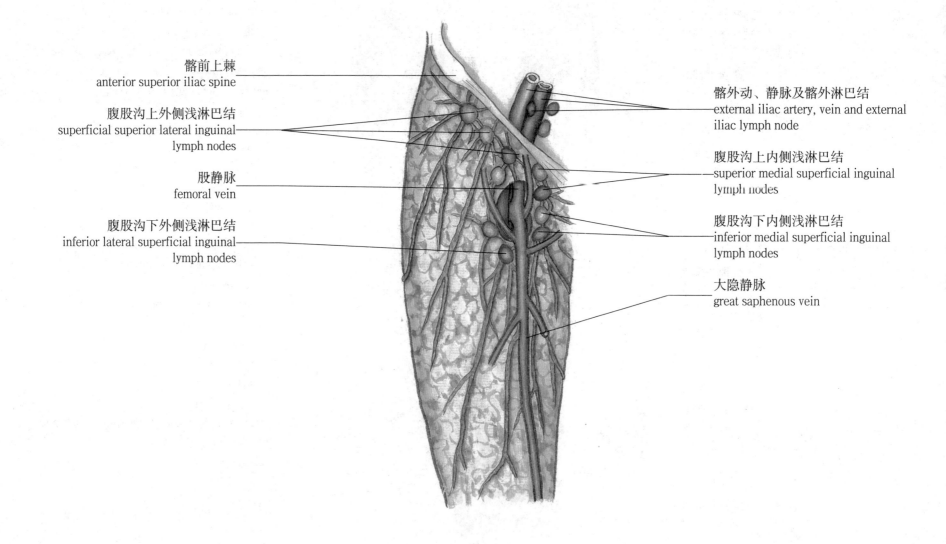

图 4-8　腹股沟浅淋巴结
Superficial inguinal lymph nodes

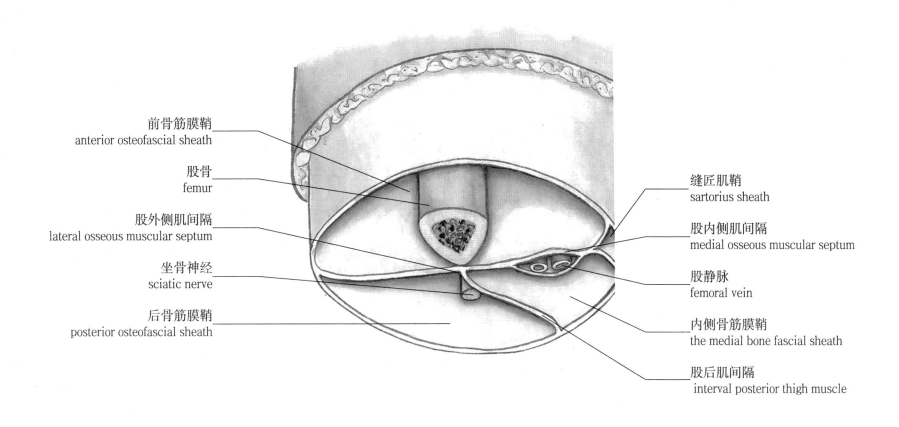

前骨筋膜鞘
anterior osteofascial sheath

股骨
femur

股外侧肌间隔
lateral osseous muscular septum

坐骨神经
sciatic nerve

后骨筋膜鞘
posterior osteofascial sheath

缝匠肌鞘
sartorius sheath

股内侧肌间隔
medial osseous muscular septum

股静脉
femoral vein

内侧骨筋膜鞘
the medial bone fascial sheath

股后肌间隔
interval posterior thigh muscle

图 4-9 股骨中部骨筋膜鞘
Osteofascial sheath of middle femur

腹股沟韧带
inguinal ligament

髂腰肌
lliopsoas muscle

股神经
femoral nerve

髂耻弓
iliopectineal arch

耻骨梳韧带
pectinate ligament

髋臼
acetabulum

股动脉
arteria femoralis

股静脉
femoral vein

股环
annulus femoralis

腔隙韧带
lacunar ligament

耻骨肌
pectineus muscle

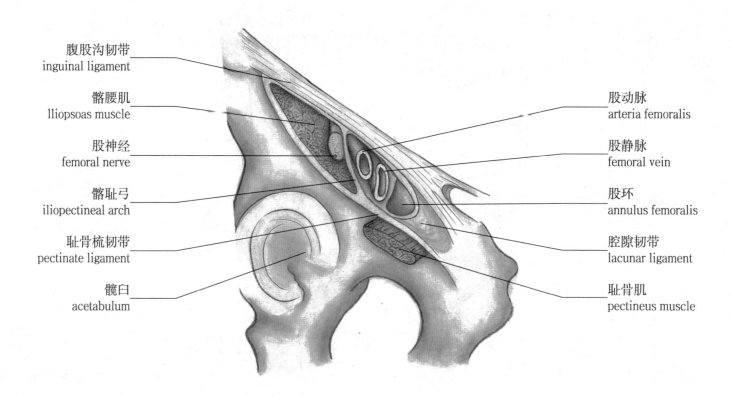

图 4-10　肌腔隙、血管腔隙
Muscle space, Vascular lacuna space

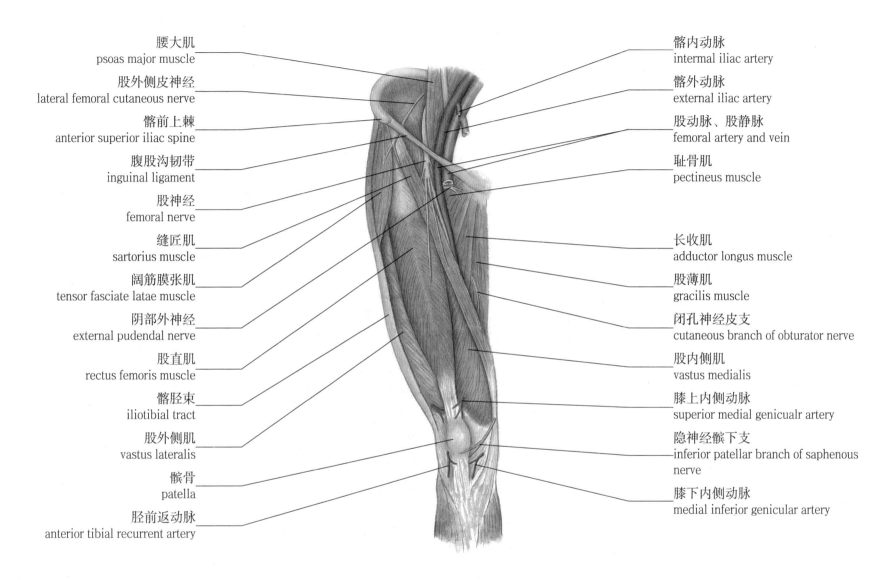

腰大肌
psoas major muscle

股外侧皮神经
lateral femoral cutaneous nerve

髂前上棘
anterior superior iliac spine

腹股沟韧带
inguinal ligament

股神经
femoral nerve

缝匠肌
sartorius muscle

阔筋膜张肌
tensor fasciate latae muscle

阴部外神经
external pudendal nerve

股直肌
rectus femoris muscle

髂胫束
iliotibial tract

股外侧肌
vastus lateralis

髌骨
patella

胫前返动脉
anterior tibial recurrent artery

髂内动脉
intermal iliac artery

髂外动脉
external iliac artery

股动脉、股静脉
femoral artery and vein

耻骨肌
pectineus muscle

长收肌
adductor longus muscle

股薄肌
gracilis muscle

闭孔神经皮支
cutaneous branch of obturator nerve

股内侧肌
vastus medialis

膝上内侧动脉
superior medial genicualr artery

隐神经髌下支
inferior patellar branch of saphenous nerve

膝下内侧动脉
medial inferior genicular artery

图 4-11 大腿前群肌、神经和血管
Anterior thigh muscles, nerves and blood vessels

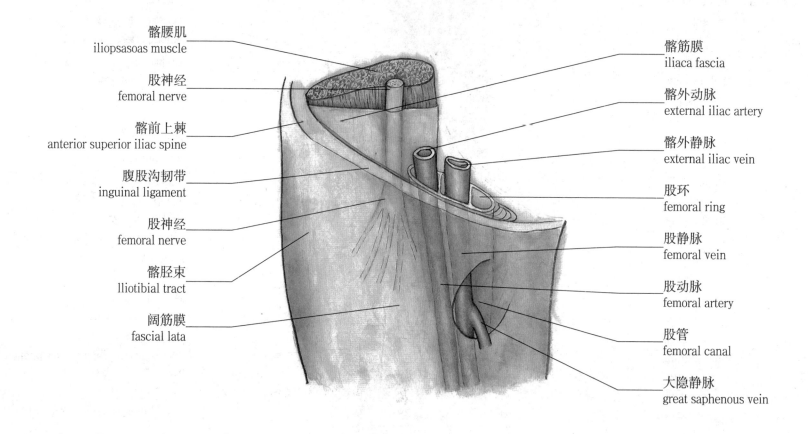

髂腰肌
iliopsasoas muscle

股神经
femoral nerve

髂前上棘
anterior superior iliac spine

腹股沟韧带
inguinal ligament

股神经
femoral nerve

髂胫束
lliotibial tract

阔筋膜
fascial lata

髂筋膜
iliaca fascia

髂外动脉
external iliac artery

髂外静脉
external iliac vein

股环
femoral ring

股静脉
femoral vein

股动脉
femoral artery

股管
femoral canal

大隐静脉
great saphenous vein

图 4-12　股鞘与股管
Femoral sheath and femoral canal

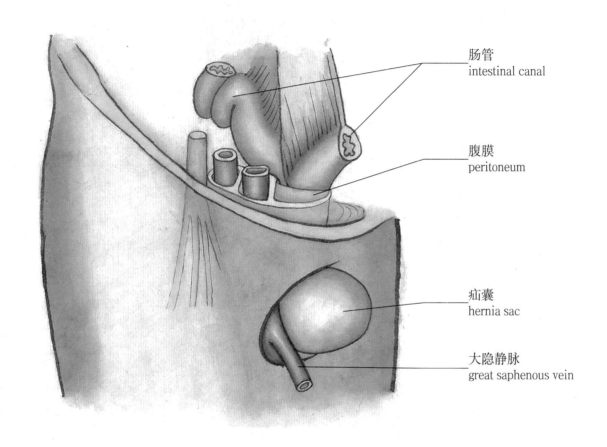

肠管
intestinal canal

腹膜
peritoneum

疝囊
hernia sac

大隐静脉
great saphenous vein

图 4-13 股疝
Femoral hernia

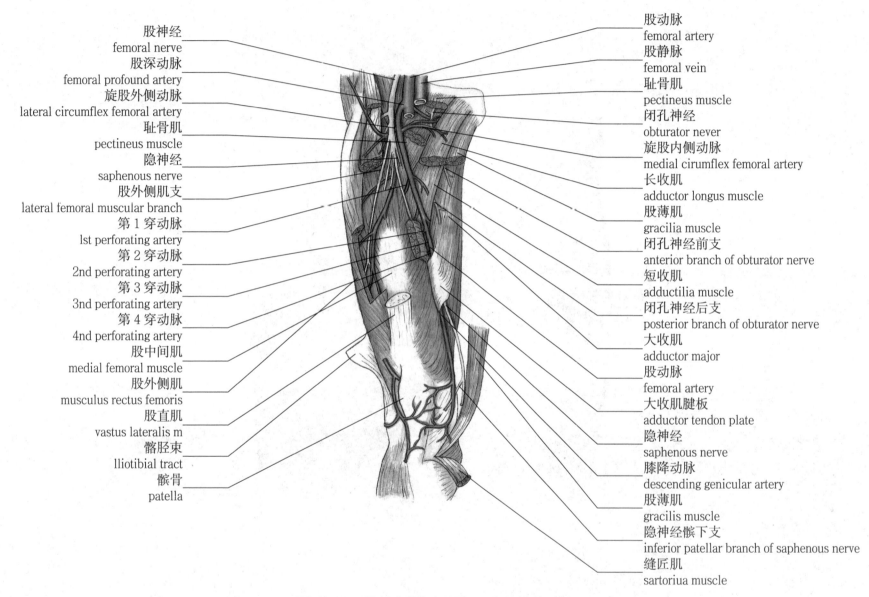

股神经
femoral nerve

股深动脉
femoral profound artery

旋股外侧动脉
lateral circumflex femoral artery

耻骨肌
pectineus muscle

隐神经
saphenous nerve

股外侧肌支
lateral femoral muscular branch

第1穿动脉
lst perforating artery

第2穿动脉
2nd perforating artery

第3穿动脉
3nd perforating artery

第4穿动脉
4nd perforating artery

股中间肌
medial femoral muscle

股外侧肌
musculus rectus femoris

股直肌
vastus lateralis m

髂胫束
lliotibial tract

髌骨
patella

股动脉
femoral artery

股静脉
femoral vein

耻骨肌
pectineus muscle

闭孔神经
obturator never

旋股内侧动脉
medial cirumflex femoral artery

长收肌
adductor longus muscle

股薄肌
gracilia muscle

闭孔神经前支
anterior branch of obturator nerve

短收肌
adductilia muscle

闭孔神经后支
posterior branch of obturator nerve

大收肌
adductor major

股动脉
femoral artery

大收肌腱板
adductor tendon plate

隐神经
saphenous nerve

膝降动脉
descending genicular artery

股薄肌
gracilis muscle

隐神经髌下支
inferior patellar branch of saphenous nerve

缝匠肌
sartoriua muscle

图 4-14 股前内侧区深层肌及血管神经
Deep muscle, blood vessel and nerve of anteromedial femoral region

臀中肌
gluteus medius
臀小肌
gluteus minimus
臀大肌
gluteus maximus
臀上神经
superior gluteal nerve
阴部内动脉及阴部神经
internal pudendal artery and nerve
坐骨结节
ischial tubercle
股后皮神经
posterior cutaneous nerve
坐骨神经
sciatic nerve
大收肌
adductor major
股薄肌
gracilia muscle
腘动脉
popliteal artery
胫神经
tibial nerve
膝上内侧动脉
medial superior genicular artery
半腱肌、半膜肌
semitendinosus, semimembranous
muscle
膝下内侧动脉
medial inferior genicular artery

梨状肌
piriformis muscle
臀下动脉
inferior gluteal artery
闭孔内肌腱及上、下孖肌
obturator tendon and superior and
inferior margin muscle
大转子
grealter trochanter
股方肌
quadratus femoris
第 1 穿动脉
1td perforating artery
第 2 穿动脉
2td perforating artery
第 3 穿动脉
3td perforating artery
髂胫束
lliotbial tract
第 4 穿动脉
4th perfrating artery
股二头肌短头
short heads of biceps femoris muscle
腓总神经
common peroneal nerve
膝上外侧动脉
superior lateral genicnlar nerve
膝中动脉
middle genicular artery
胫神经肌支
muscular branch of femoral nerve
膝下外侧动脉
inferior lateral genicular artery
腓肠内侧皮神经
medial sural cutaneous nerve
腓肠外侧皮神经
lateral sural cutaneous nerve

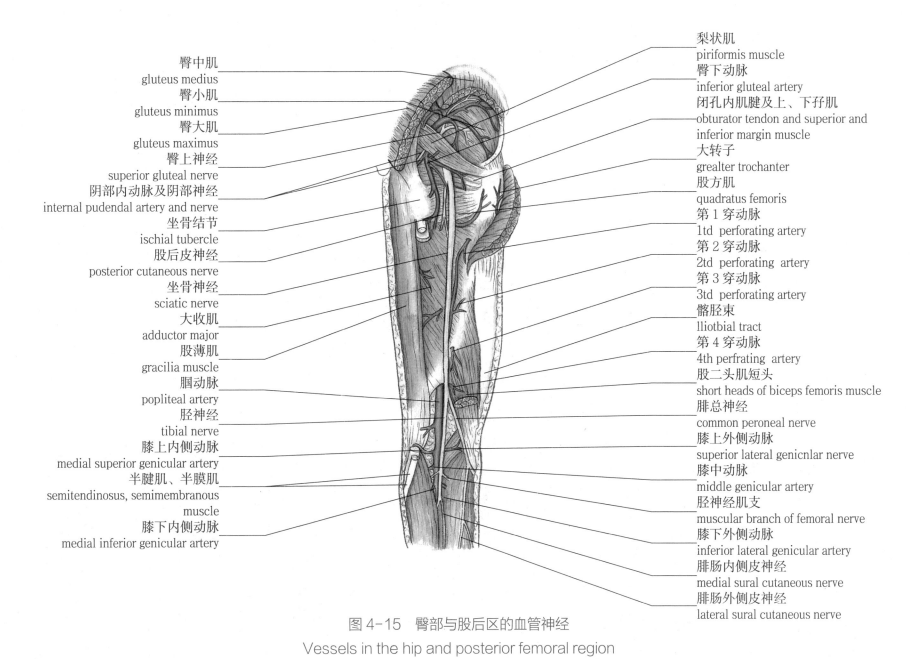

图 4-15 臀部与股后区的血管神经

Vessels in the hip and posterior femoral region

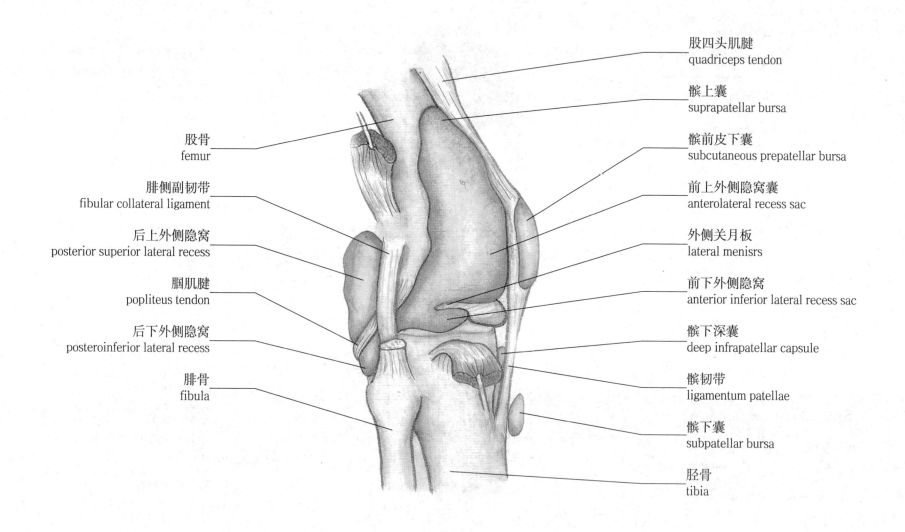

股四头肌腱
quadriceps tendon

髌上囊
suprapatellar bursa

股骨
femur

髌前皮下囊
subcutaneous prepatellar bursa

腓侧副韧带
fibular collateral ligament

前上外侧隐窝囊
anterolateral recess sac

后上外侧隐窝
posterior superior lateral recess

外侧关月板
lateral menisrs

腘肌腱
popliteus tendon

前下外侧隐窝
anterior inferior lateral recess sac

后下外侧隐窝
posteroinferior lateral recess

髌下深囊
deep infrapatellar capsule

腓骨
fibula

髌韧带
ligamentum patellae

髌下囊
subpatellar bursa

胫骨
tibia

图 4-16　膝关节滑液囊
Synovial sac of knee joint

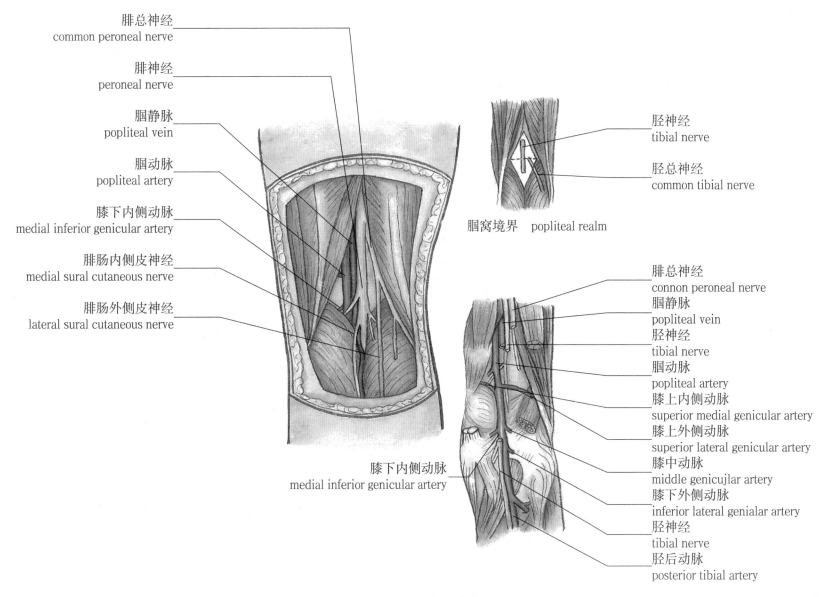

腓总神经
common peroneal nerve

腓神经
peroneal nerve

腘静脉
popliteal vein

腘动脉
popliteal artery

膝下内侧动脉
medial inferior genicular artery

腓肠内侧皮神经
medial sural cutaneous nerve

腓肠外侧皮神经
lateral sural cutaneous nerve

胫神经
tibial nerve

胫总神经
common tibial nerve

腘窝境界　popliteal realm

腓总神经
connon peroneal nerve

腘静脉
popliteal vein

胫神经
tibial nerve

腘动脉
popliteal artery

膝上内侧动脉
superior medial genicular artery

膝上外侧动脉
superior lateral genicular artery

膝中动脉
middle genicujlar artery

膝下外侧动脉
inferior lateral genialar artery

胫神经
tibial nerve

胫后动脉
posterior tibial artery

膝下内侧动脉
medial inferior genicular artery

图 4-17　腘窝及内容
Popliteal fossa and content

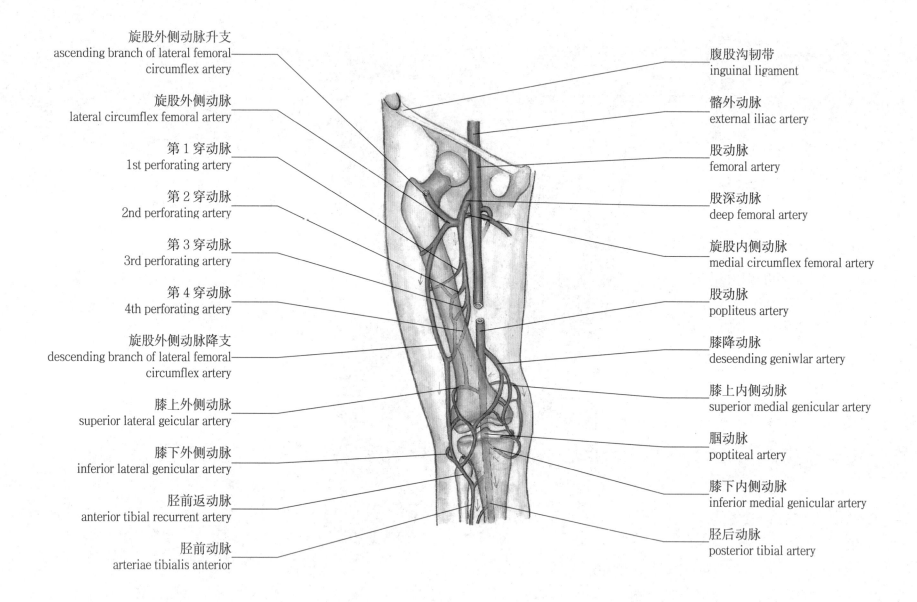

旋股外侧动脉升支
ascending branch of lateral femoral
circumflex artery

旋股外侧动脉
lateral circumflex femoral artery

第 1 穿动脉
1st perforating artery

第 2 穿动脉
2nd perforating artery

第 3 穿动脉
3rd perforating artery

第 4 穿动脉
4th perforating artery

旋股外侧动脉降支
descending branch of lateral femoral
circumflex artery

膝上外侧动脉
superior lateral geicular artery

膝下外侧动脉
inferior lateral genicular artery

胫前返动脉
anterior tibial recurrent artery

胫前动脉
arteriae tibialis anterior

腹股沟韧带
inguinal ligament

髂外动脉
external iliac artery

股动脉
femoral artery

股深动脉
deep femoral artery

旋股内侧动脉
medial circumflex femoral artery

股动脉
popliteus artery

膝降动脉
deseending geniwlar artery

膝上内侧动脉
superior medial genicular artery

腘动脉
poptiteal artery

膝下内侧动脉
inferior medial genicular artery

胫后动脉
posterior tibial artery

图 4-18 膝关节动脉网
Arterial network of knee joint

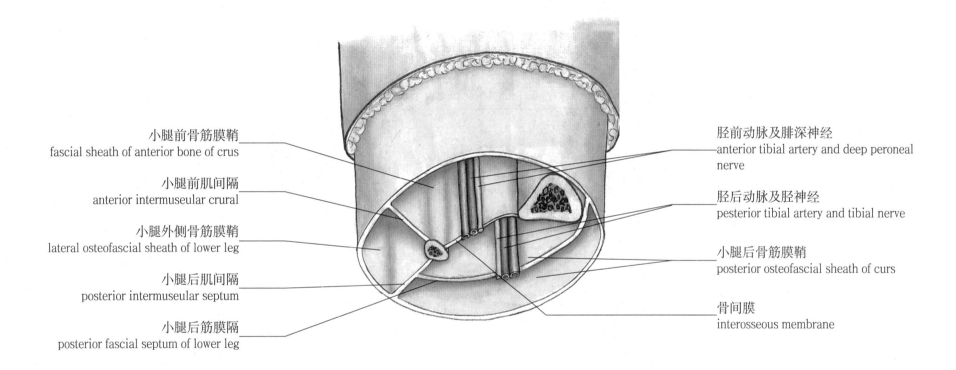

小腿前骨筋膜鞘
fascial sheath of anterior bone of crus

小腿前肌间隔
anterior intermuseular crural

小腿外侧骨筋膜鞘
lateral osteofascial sheath of lower leg

小腿后肌间隔
posterior intermuseular septum

小腿后筋膜隔
posterior fascial septum of lower leg

胫前动脉及腓深神经
anterior tibial artery and deep peroneal nerve

胫后动脉及胫神经
pesterior tibial artery and tibial nerve

小腿后骨筋膜鞘
posterior osteofascial sheath of curs

骨间膜
interosseous membrane

图 4-19 小腿中部骨筋膜鞘
Osteofascial sheath of curs

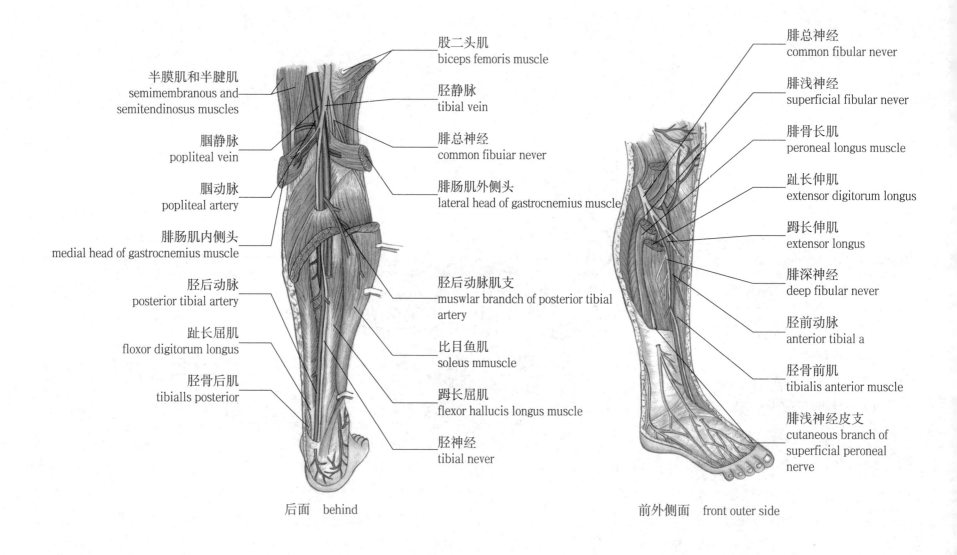

半膜肌和半腱肌
semimembranous and
semitendinosus muscles

腘静脉
popliteal vein

腘动脉
popliteal artery

腓肠肌内侧头
medial head of gastrocnemius muscle

胫后动脉
posterior tibial artery

趾长屈肌
floxor digitorum longus

胫骨后肌
tibialls posterior

股二头肌
biceps femoris muscle

胫静脉
tibial vein

腓总神经
common fibuiar never

腓肠肌外侧头
lateral head of gastrocnemius muscle

胫后动脉肌支
muswlar brandch of posterior tibial
artery

比目鱼肌
soleus mmuscle

蹈长屈肌
flexor hallucis longus muscle

胫神经
tibial never

腓总神经
common fibular never

腓浅神经
superficial fibular never

腓骨长肌
peroneal longus muscle

趾长伸肌
extensor digitorum longus

蹈长伸肌
extensor longus

腓深神经
deep fibular never

胫前动脉
anterior tibial a

胫骨前肌
tibialis anterior muscle

腓浅神经皮支
cutaneous branch of
superficial peroneal
nerve

后面　behind

前外侧面　front outer side

图 4-20　小腿的血管神经
Blood vessels and nerves of lower leg

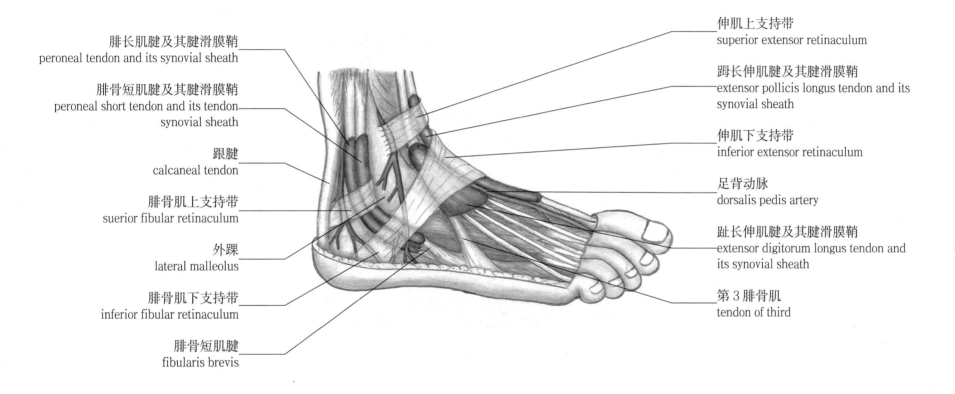

腓长肌腱及其腱滑膜鞘
peroneal tendon and its synovial sheath

腓骨短肌腱及其腱滑膜鞘
peroneal short tendon and its tendon
synovial sheath

跟腱
calcaneal tendon

腓骨肌上支持带
suerior fibular retinaculum

外踝
lateral malleolus

腓骨肌下支持带
inferior fibular retinaculum

腓骨短肌腱
fibularis brevis

伸肌上支持带
superior extensor retinaculum

蹈长伸肌腱及其腱滑膜鞘
extensor pollicis longus tendon and its
synovial sheath

伸肌下支持带
inferior extensor retinaculum

足背动脉
dorsalis pedis artery

趾长伸肌腱及其腱滑膜鞘
extensor digitorum longus tendon and
its synovial sheath

第 3 腓骨肌
tendon of third

图 4-21　小腿肌支持带及腱鞘（外侧面）
Calf muscle retinaculum and tendon sheath（outer side）

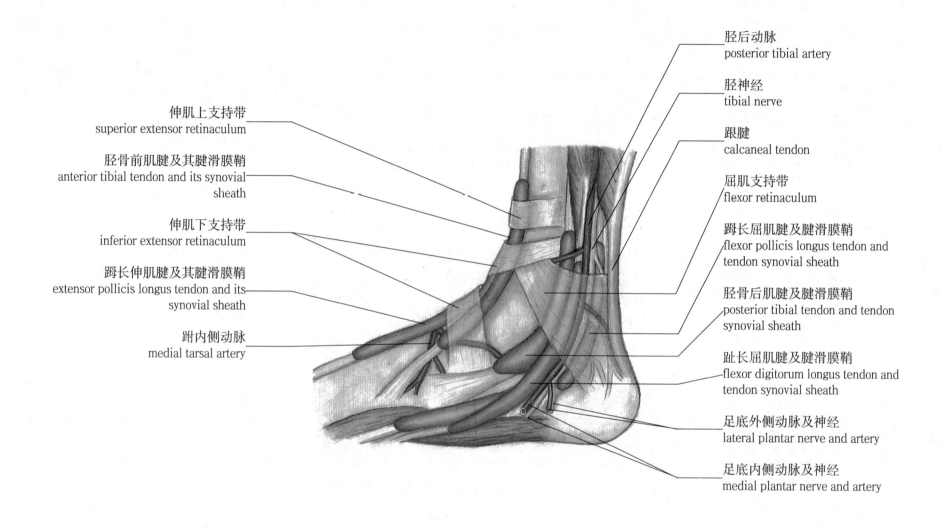

伸肌上支持带
superior extensor retinaculum

胫骨前肌腱及其腱滑膜鞘
anterior tibial tendon and its synovial sheath

伸肌下支持带
inferior extensor retinaculum

踇长伸肌腱及其腱滑膜鞘
extensor pollicis longus tendon and its synovial sheath

跗内侧动脉
medial tarsal artery

胫后动脉
posterior tibial artery

胫神经
tibial nerve

跟腱
calcaneal tendon

屈肌支持带
flexor retinaculum

踇长屈肌腱及腱滑膜鞘
flexor pollicis longus tendon and tendon synovial sheath

胫骨后肌腱及腱滑膜鞘
posterior tibial tendon and tendon synovial sheath

趾长屈肌腱及腱滑膜鞘
flexor digitorum longus tendon and tendon synovial sheath

足底外侧动脉及神经
lateral plantar nerve and artery

足底内侧动脉及神经
medial plantar nerve and artery

图 4-22 小腿肌支持带及腱鞘（内侧面）
Calf muscle retinaculum and tendon sheath （medial surface）

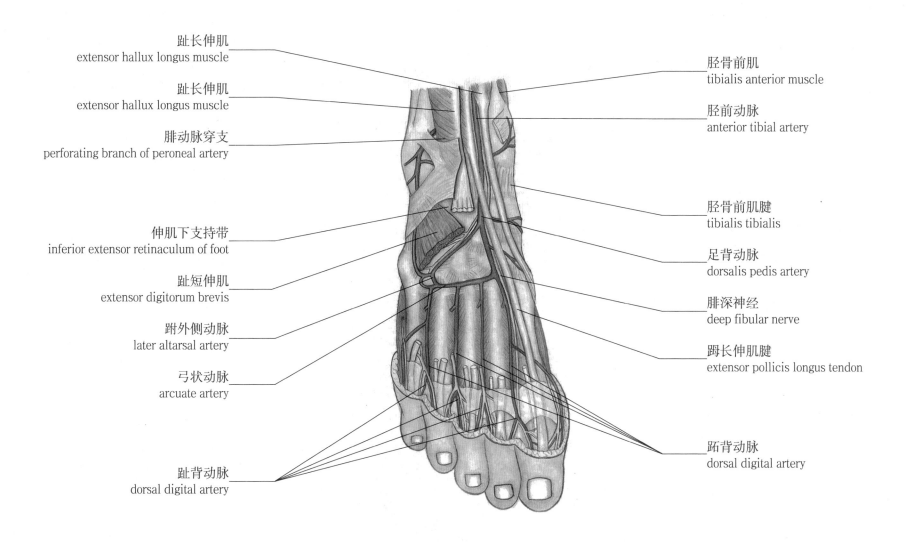

趾长伸肌
extensor hallux longus muscle

趾长伸肌
extensor hallux longus muscle

腓动脉穿支
perforating branch of peroneal artery

伸肌下支持带
inferior extensor retinaculum of foot

趾短伸肌
extensor digitorum brevis

跗外侧动脉
later altarsal artery

弓状动脉
arcuate artery

趾背动脉
dorsal digital artery

胫骨前肌
tibialis anterior muscle

胫前动脉
anterior tibial artery

胫骨前肌腱
tibialis tibialis

足背动脉
dorsalis pedis artery

腓深神经
deep fibular nerve

蹈长伸肌腱
extensor pollicis longus tendon

跖背动脉
dorsal digital artery

图 4-23 踝前区及足背
Premalleolar area and dorsum of foot

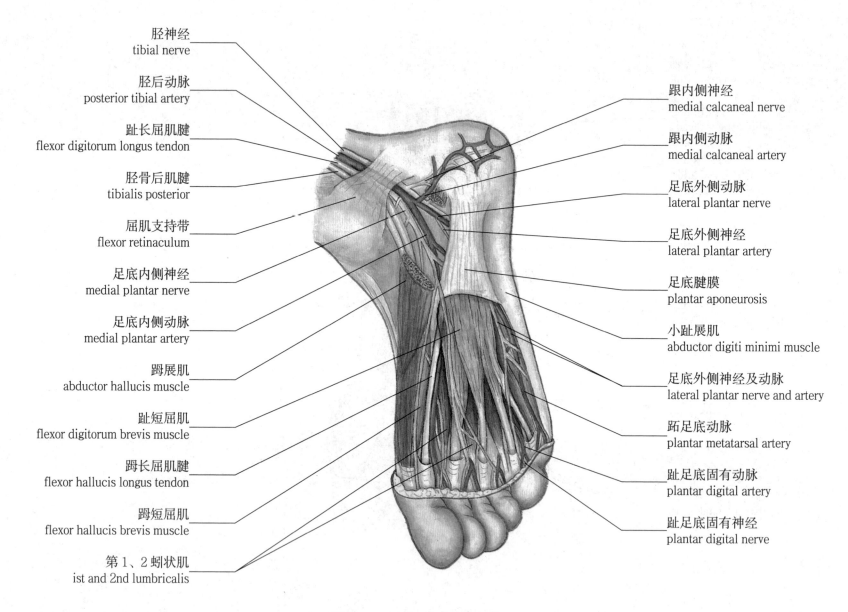

胫神经
tibial nerve

胫后动脉
posterior tibial artery

趾长屈肌腱
flexor digitorum longus tendon

胫骨后肌腱
tibialis posterior

屈肌支持带
flexor retinaculum

足底内侧神经
medial plantar nerve

足底内侧动脉
medial plantar artery

踇展肌
abductor hallucis muscle

趾短屈肌
flexor digitorum brevis muscle

踇长屈肌腱
flexor hallucis longus tendon

踇短屈肌
flexor hallucis brevis muscle

第 1、2 蚓状肌
ist and 2nd lumbricalis

跟内侧神经
medial calcaneal nerve

跟内侧动脉
medial calcaneal artery

足底外侧动脉
lateral plantar nerve

足底外侧神经
lateral plantar artery

足底腱膜
plantar aponeurosis

小趾展肌
abductor digiti minimi muscle

足底外侧神经及动脉
lateral plantar nerve and artery

跖足底动脉
plantar metatarsal artery

趾足底固有动脉
plantar digital artery

趾足底固有神经
plantar digital nerve

图 4-24 踝后区内侧面及足底
Medial side of posterior ankle and sole

伸肌上支持带
superior extensor retinaculum

腓骨短肌
peroneal short muscle

腓动脉末支
terminal branch of peroneal artery

腓骨肌上支持带
superior fibular retinaeulun

腓骨长肌腱
peroneus longus tendon

腓骨肌下支持带
subperoneal retinaculum

第 3 腓骨肌腱
third peroneal tendon

胫骨前肌
tibialis anterior anterior tibial muscle

踇长伸肌
extensor hallucis longus muscle

趾长伸肌
extensor digitorum longus muscle

伸肌下支持带
subextensor retinaculum

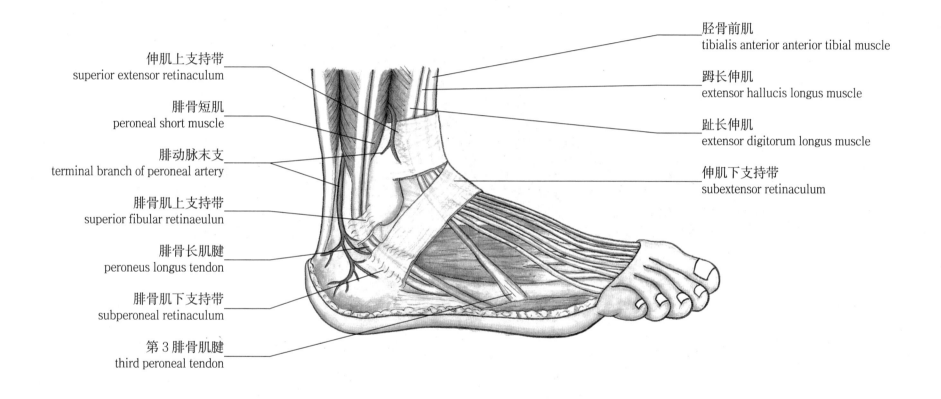

图 4-25 踝与足背外侧面
Lateral surface of ankle and dorsum of foot

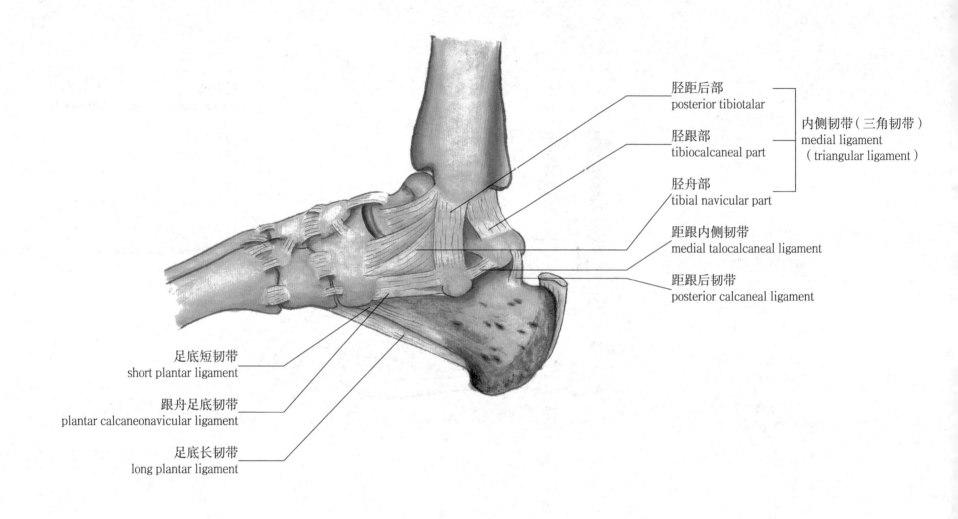

胫距后部
posterior tibiotalar

胫跟部
tibiocalcaneal part

胫舟部
tibial navicular part

内侧韧带（三角韧带）
medial ligament
（triangular ligament）

距跟内侧韧带
medial talocalcaneal ligament

距跟后韧带
posterior calcaneal ligament

足底短韧带
short plantar ligament

跟舟足底韧带
plantar calcaneonavicular ligament

足底长韧带
long plantar ligament

图 4-26　足的韧带（内侧面观）
Ligaments of foot（medial surface）

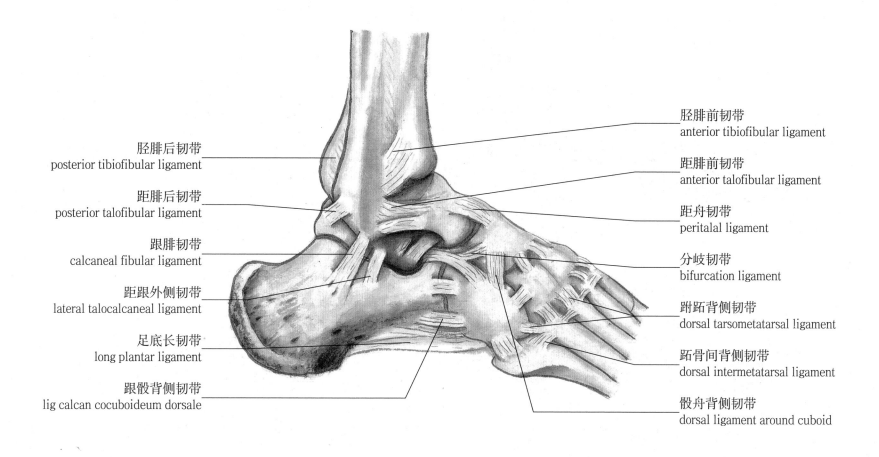

胫腓后韧带
posterior tibiofibular ligament

距腓后韧带
posterior talofibular ligament

跟腓韧带
calcaneal fibular ligament

距跟外侧韧带
lateral talocalcaneal ligament

足底长韧带
long plantar ligament

跟骰背侧韧带
lig calcan cocuboideum dorsale

胫腓前韧带
anterior tibiofibular ligament

距腓前韧带
anterior talofibular ligament

距舟韧带
peritalal ligament

分岐韧带
bifurcation ligament

跗跖背侧韧带
dorsal tarsometatarsal ligament

跖骨间背侧韧带
dorsal intermetatarsal ligament

骰舟背侧韧带
dorsal ligament around cuboid

图 4-27　足的韧带（外侧面观）
Ligaments of foot（outer side）

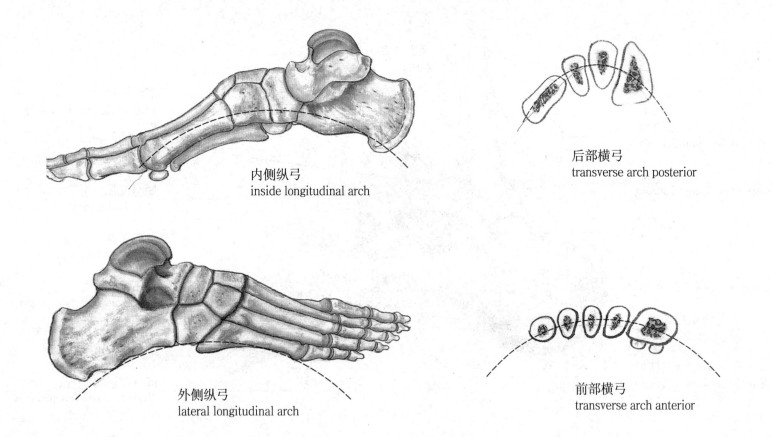

内侧纵弓
inside longitudinal arch

后部横弓
transverse arch posterior

外侧纵弓
lateral longitudinal arch

前部横弓
transverse arch anterior

图 4-28 足弓
Arch of foot

第五章

胸部

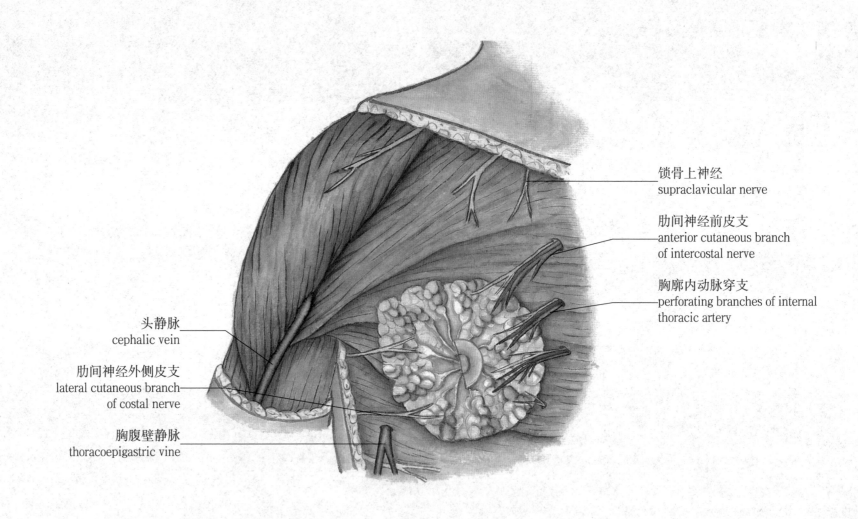

锁骨上神经
supraclavicular nerve

肋间神经前皮支
anterior cutaneous branch
of intercostal nerve

胸廓内动脉穿支
perforating branches of internal
thoracic artery

头静脉
cephalic vein

肋间神经外侧皮支
lateral cutaneous branch
of costal nerve

胸腹壁静脉
thoracoepigastric vine

图 5-1　胸前、外侧区的浅血管和皮神经
Superficial vessels and cutaneous nerves in the anterior and lateral regions of the chest

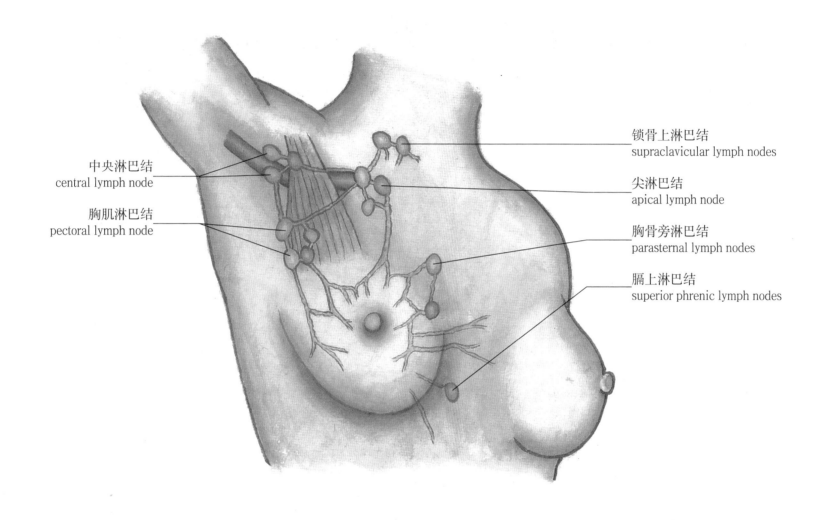

锁骨上淋巴结
supraclavicular lymph nodes

中央淋巴结
central lymph node

尖淋巴结
apical lymph node

胸肌淋巴结
pectoral lymph node

胸骨旁淋巴结
parasternal lymph nodes

膈上淋巴结
superior phrenic lymph nodes

图 5-2　乳房的淋巴回流
lymphatic reflux of breast

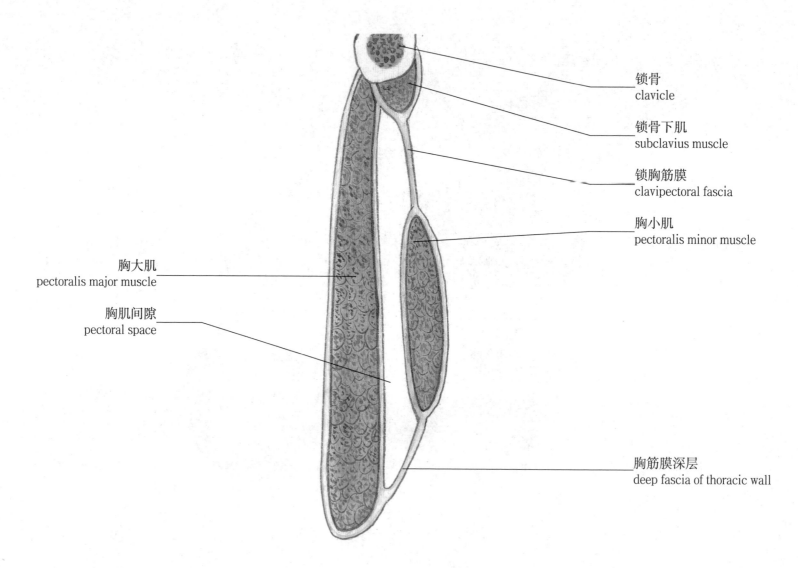

锁骨
clavicle

锁骨下肌
subclavius muscle

锁胸筋膜
clavipectoral fascia

胸小肌
pectoralis minor muscle

胸大肌
pectoralis major muscle

胸肌间隙
pectoral space

胸筋膜深层
deep fascia of thoracic wall

图 5-3　胸前区深筋膜
Deep fascia of precordial region

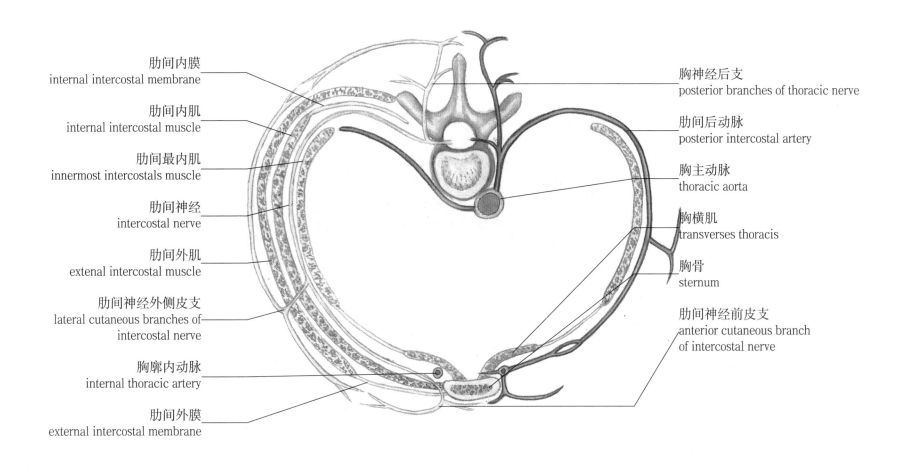

肋间内膜
internal intercostal membrane

肋间内肌
internal intercostal muscle

肋间最内肌
innermost intercostals muscle

肋间神经
intercostal nerve

肋间外肌
extenal intercostal muscle

肋间神经外侧皮支
lateral cutaneous branches of
intercostal nerve

胸廓内动脉
internal thoracic artery

肋间外膜
external intercostal membrane

胸神经后支
posterior branches of thoracic nerve

肋间后动脉
posterior intercostal artery

胸主动脉
thoracic aorta

胸横肌
transverses thoracis

胸骨
sternum

肋间神经前皮支
anterior cutaneous branch
of intercostal nerve

图 5-4　肋间后动脉和肋间神经
Posterior intercostal artery and intercostal nerve

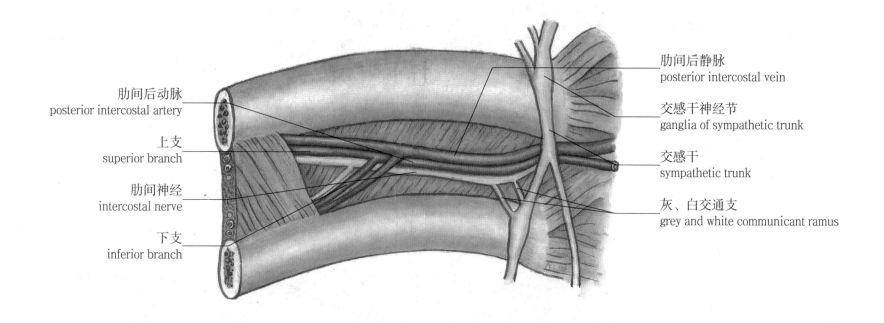

肋间后动脉
posterior intercostal artery

肋间后静脉
posterior intercostal vein

交感干神经节
ganglia of sympathetic trunk

上支
superior branch

交感干
sympathetic trunk

肋间神经
intercostal nerve

灰、白交通支
grey and white communicant ramus

下支
inferior branch

图 5-5　肋间后血管、肋间神经和胸交感干
Posterior intercostal vessels, intercostal nerves and thoracic sympathetic trunk

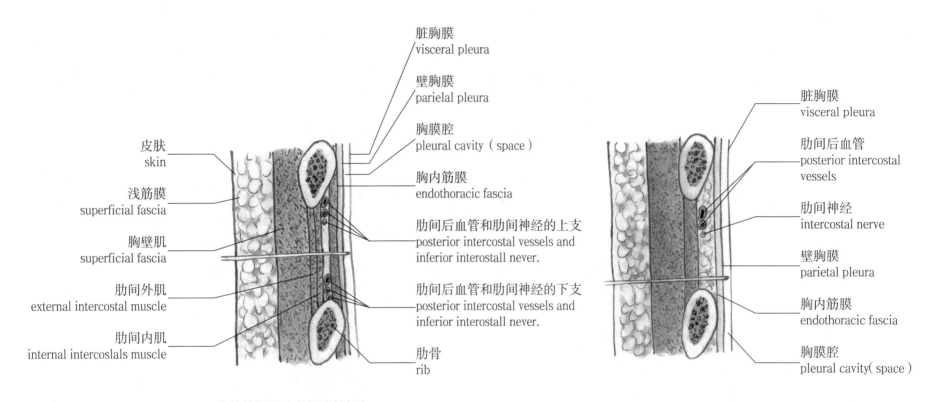

脏胸膜
visceral pleura

壁胸膜
parielal pleura

胸膜腔
pleural cavity（space）

胸内筋膜
endothoracic fascia

皮肤
skin

浅筋膜
superficial fascia

胸壁肌
superficial fascia

肋间外肌
external intercostal muscle

肋间内肌
internal intercoslals muscle

肋间后血管和肋间神经的上支
posterior intercostal vessels and inferior interostall never.

肋间后血管和肋间神经的下支
posterior intercostal vessels and inferior interostall never.

肋骨
rib

脏胸膜
visceral pleura

肋间后血管
posterior intercostal vessels

肋间神经
intercostal nerve

壁胸膜
parietal pleura

胸内筋膜
endothoracic fascia

胸膜腔
pleural cavity（space）

胸前外侧壁（肩押线外侧）
anterolateral chest wall（lateral scapular line）

胸后壁（肩胛线内侧）
posterior chest wall（medial scapular line）

图 5-6　胸壁层次及胸膜腔穿刺部位
Level of chest wall and puncture site of pleural cavity

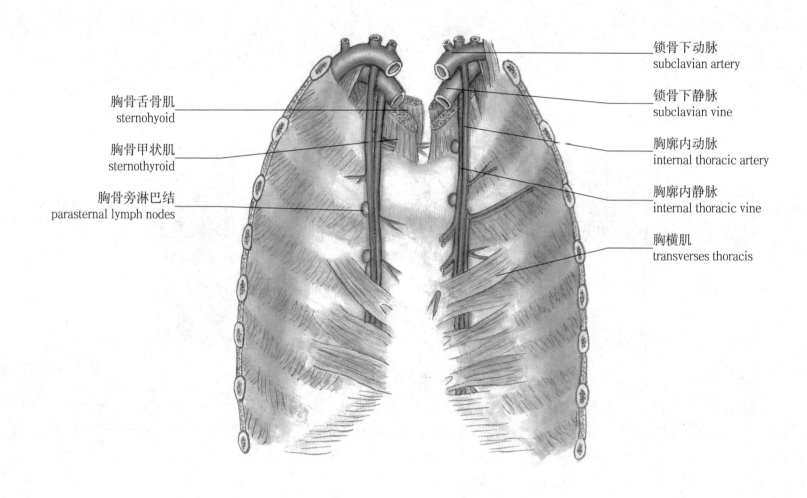

锁骨下动脉
subclavian artery

锁骨下静脉
subclavian vine

胸廓内动脉
internal thoracic artery

胸廓内静脉
internal thoracic vine

胸横肌
transverses thoracis

胸骨舌骨肌
sternohyoid

胸骨甲状肌
sternothyroid

胸骨旁淋巴结
parasternal lymph nodes

图 5-7 胸廓内血管和胸骨旁淋巴结
Intrathoracic vessels and parasternal lymph nodes

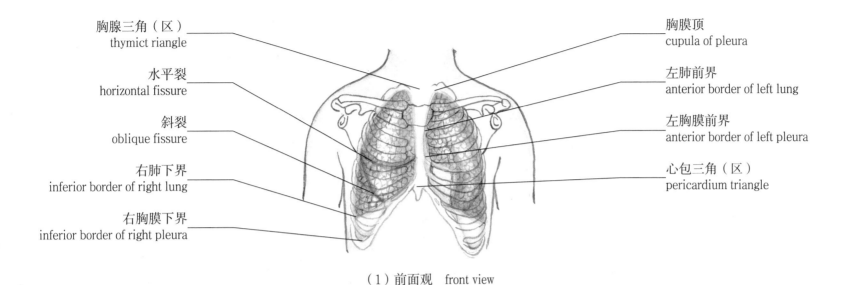

胸腺三角（区）
thymict riangle

水平裂
horizontal fissure

斜裂
oblique fissure

右肺下界
inferior border of right lung

右胸膜下界
inferior border of right pleura

胸膜顶
cupula of pleura

左肺前界
anterior border of left lung

左胸膜前界
anterior border of left pleura

心包三角（区）
pericardium triangle

（1）前面观　front view

胸膜顶
cupula pleura

斜裂
oblique fissure

左肺下界
inferior border of left lung

左胸膜下界
inferior border of left pleura

（2）左侧面观　leftsideview

图 5-8-1　胸膜和肺的体表投影
Body surface projection of chest model and lung

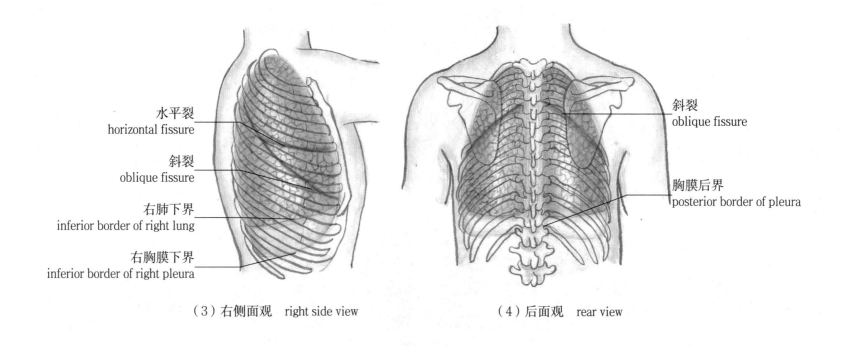

水平裂
horizontal fissure

斜裂
oblique fissure

右肺下界
inferior border of right lung

右胸膜下界
inferior border of right pleura

斜裂
oblique fissure

胸膜后界
posterior border of pleura

（3）右侧面观　right side view

（4）后面观　rear view

图 5-8-2　胸膜和肺的体表投影
Body surface projection of chestmodel and lung

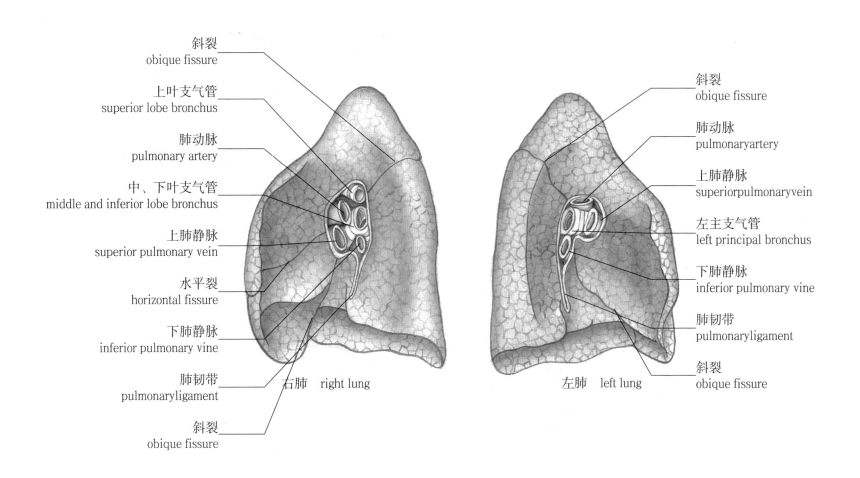

斜裂
obique fissure

上叶支气管
superior lobe bronchus

肺动脉
pulmonary artery

中、下叶支气管
middle and inferior lobe bronchus

上肺静脉
superior pulmonary vein

水平裂
horizontal fissure

下肺静脉
inferior pulmonary vine

肺韧带
pulmonaryligament

石肺　right lung

斜裂
obique fissure

斜裂
obique fissure

肺动脉
pulmonaryartery

上肺静脉
superiorpulmonaryvein

左主支气管
left principal bronchus

下肺静脉
inferior pulmonary vine

肺韧带
pulmonaryligament

斜裂
obique fissure

左肺　left lung

图 5-9　肺根的结构
Structure of lung root

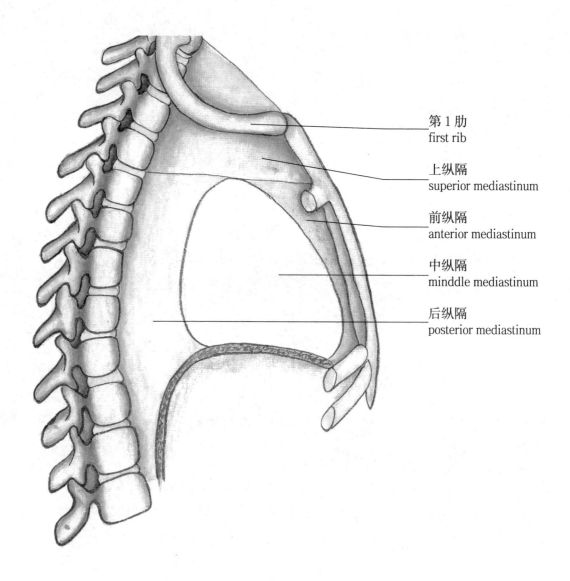

第 1 肋
first rib

上纵隔
superior mediastinum

前纵隔
anterior mediastinum

中纵隔
minddle mediastinum

后纵隔
posterior mediastinum

图 5-10　纵隔分区
Mediastinal partition

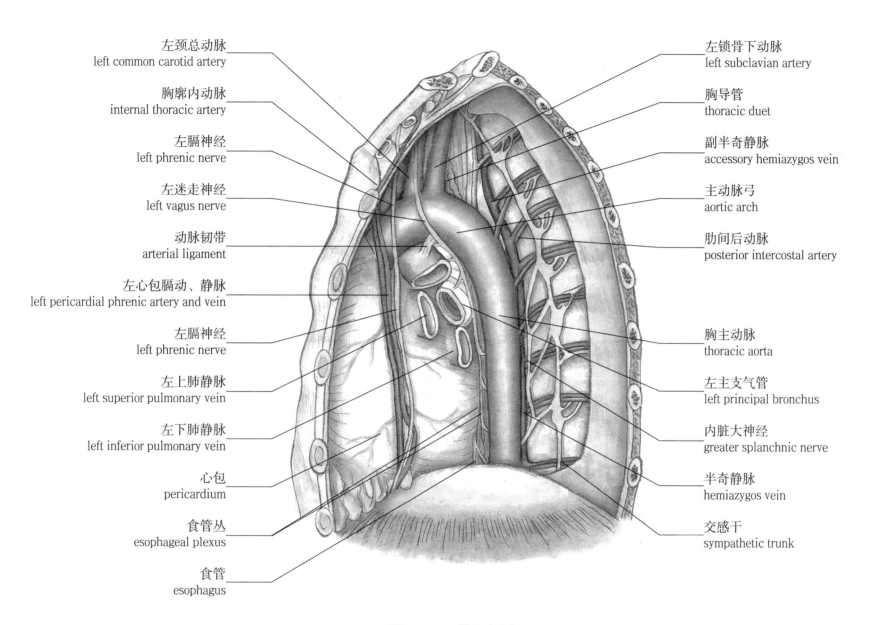

左颈总动脉
left common carotid artery

胸廓内动脉
internal thoracic artery

左膈神经
left phrenic nerve

左迷走神经
left vagus nerve

动脉韧带
arterial ligament

左心包膈动、静脉
left pericardial phrenic artery and vein

左膈神经
left phrenic nerve

左上肺静脉
left superior pulmonary vein

左下肺静脉
left inferior pulmonary vein

心包
pericardium

食管丛
esophageal plexus

食管
esophagus

左锁骨下动脉
left subclavian artery

胸导管
thoracic duet

副半奇静脉
accessory hemiazygos vein

主动脉弓
aortic arch

肋间后动脉
posterior intercostal artery

胸主动脉
thoracic aorta

左主支气管
left principal bronchus

内脏大神经
greater splanchnic nerve

半奇静脉
hemiazygos vein

交感干
sympathetic trunk

图 5-11 纵隔左侧面观
Left side view of mediastinum

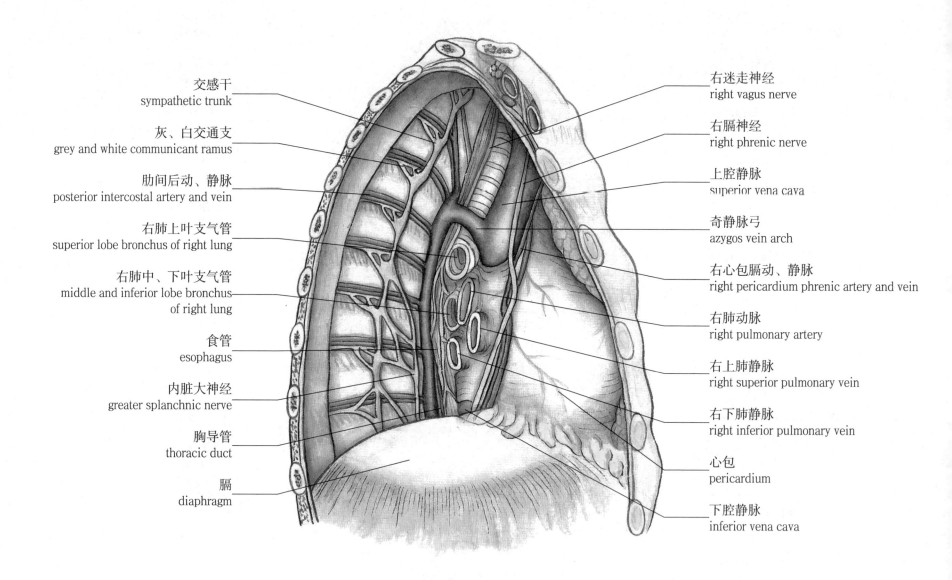

交感干
sympathetic trunk

灰、白交通支
grey and white communicant ramus

肋间后动、静脉
posterior intercostal artery and vein

右肺上叶支气管
superior lobe bronchus of right lung

右肺中、下叶支气管
middle and inferior lobe bronchus
of right lung

食管
esophagus

内脏大神经
greater splanchnic nerve

胸导管
thoracic duct

膈
diaphragm

右迷走神经
right vagus nerve

右膈神经
right phrenic nerve

上腔静脉
superior vena cava

奇静脉弓
azygos vein arch

右心包膈动、静脉
right pericardium phrenic artery and vein

右肺动脉
right pulmonary artery

右上肺静脉
right superior pulmonary vein

右下肺静脉
right inferior pulmonary vein

心包
pericardium

下腔静脉
inferior vena cava

图 5-12　纵隔右侧面观
Right side view of mediastinum

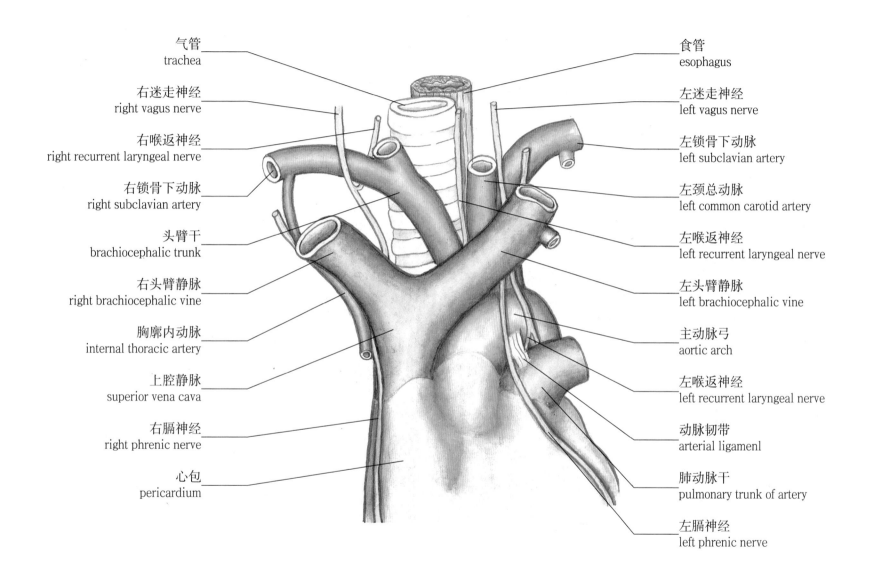

气管
trachea

食管
esophagus

右迷走神经
right vagus nerve

左迷走神经
left vagus nerve

右喉返神经
right recurrent laryngeal nerve

左锁骨下动脉
left subclavian artery

右锁骨下动脉
right subclavian artery

左颈总动脉
left common carotid artery

头臂干
brachiocephalic trunk

左喉返神经
left recurrent laryngeal nerve

右头臂静脉
right brachiocephalic vine

左头臂静脉
left brachiocephalic vine

胸廓内动脉
internal thoracic artery

主动脉弓
aortic arch

上腔静脉
superior vena cava

左喉返神经
left recurrent laryngeal nerve

右膈神经
right phrenic nerve

动脉韧带
arterial ligamenl

心包
pericardium

肺动脉干
pulmonary trunk of artery

左膈神经
left phrenic nerve

图 5-13　上纵隔的结构
Structure of upper mediastinum

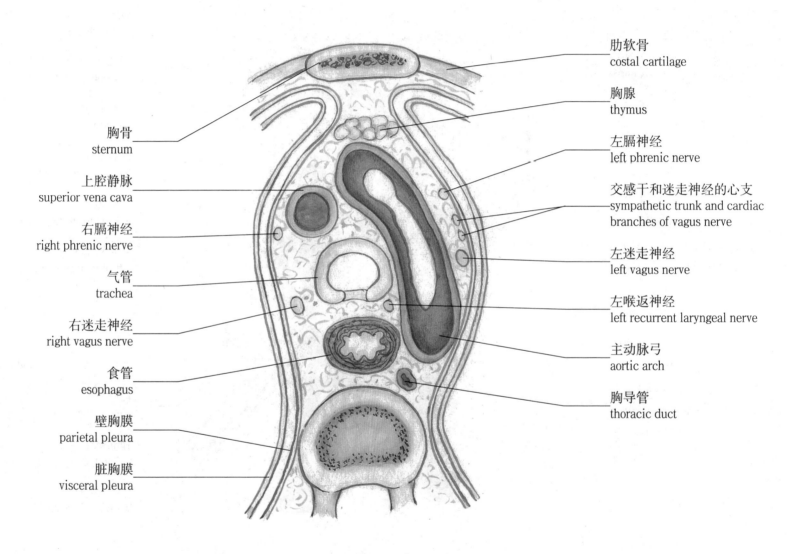

肋软骨
costal cartilage

胸腺
thymus

左膈神经
left phrenic nerve

交感干和迷走神经的心支
sympathetic trunk and cardiac
branches of vagus nerve

左迷走神经
left vagus nerve

左喉返神经
left recurrent laryngeal nerve

主动脉弓
aortic arch

胸导管
thoracic duct

胸骨
sternum

上腔静脉
superior vena cava

右膈神经
right phrenic nerve

气管
trachea

右迷走神经
right vagus nerve

食管
esophagus

壁胸膜
parietal pleura

脏胸膜
visceral pleura

图 5-14　上纵隔横断面（平第 4 胸椎）
Up per mediastinal cross section（Flat 4th thoracic vertebra）

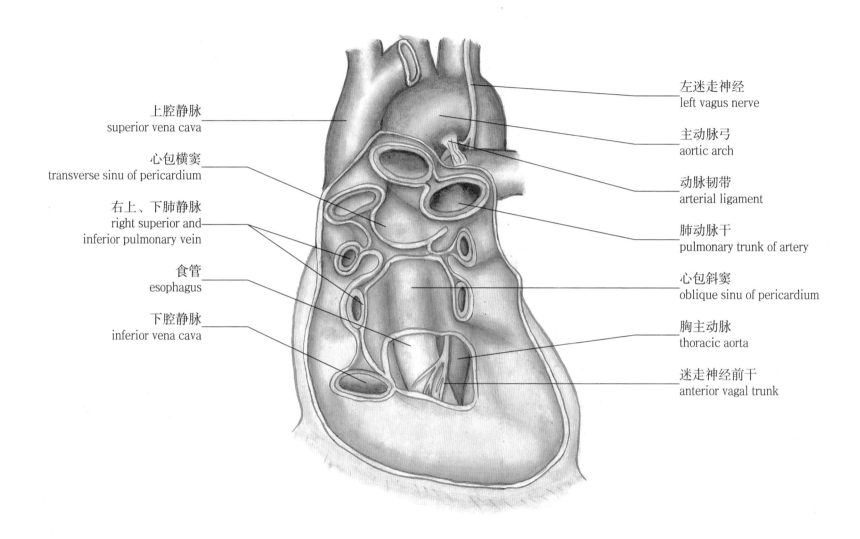

上腔静脉
superior vena cava

心包横窦
transverse sinu of pericardium

右上、下肺静脉
right superior and
inferior pulmonary vein

食管
esophagus

下腔静脉
inferior vena cava

左迷走神经
left vagus nerve

主动脉弓
aortic arch

动脉韧带
arterial ligament

肺动脉干
pulmonary trunk of artery

心包斜窦
oblique sinu of pericardium

胸主动脉
thoracic aorta

迷走神经前干
anterior vagal trunk

图 5-15 心包及心包窦
Pericardium and pericardial sinus

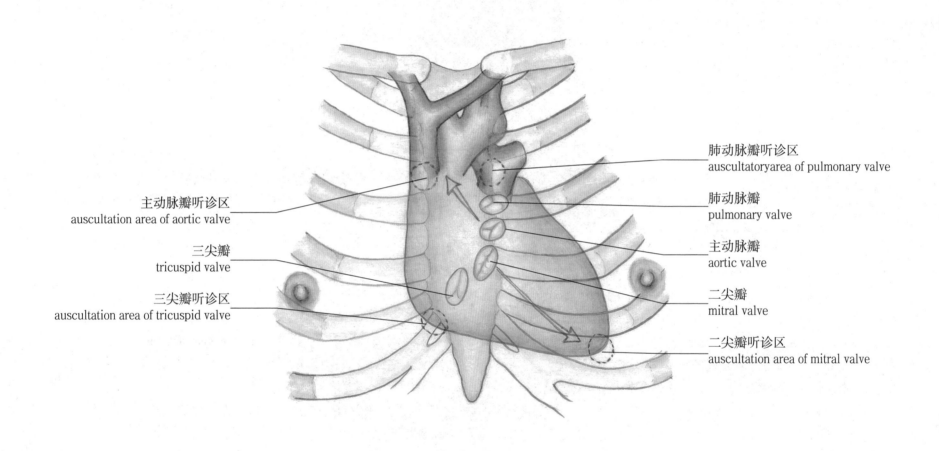

主动脉瓣听诊区
auscultation area of aortic valve

三尖瓣
tricuspid valve

三尖瓣听诊区
auscultation area of tricuspid valve

肺动脉瓣听诊区
auscultatoryarea of pulmonary valve

肺动脉瓣
pulmonary valve

主动脉瓣
aortic valve

二尖瓣
mitral valve

二尖瓣听诊区
auscultation area of mitral valve

图 5-16　心的体表投影
Body surface projection of heart

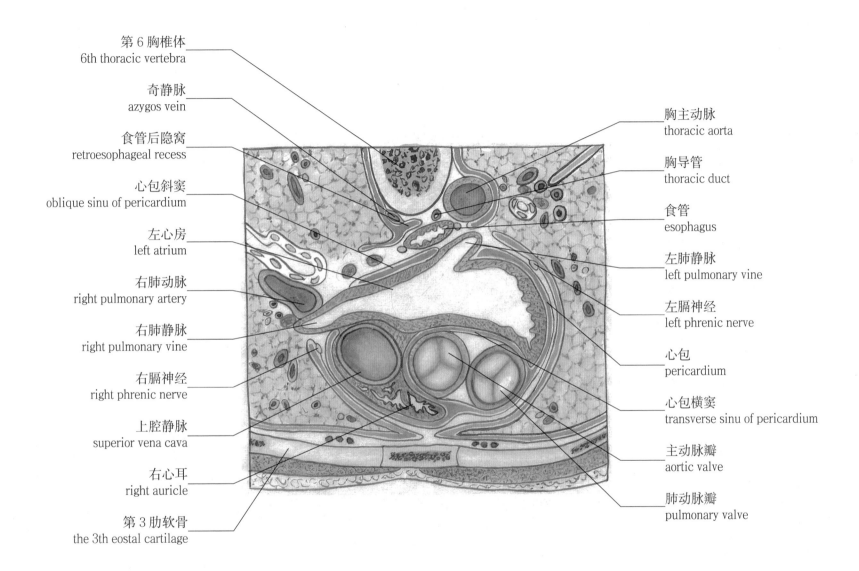

第 6 胸椎体
6th thoracic vertebra

奇静脉
azygos vein

食管后隐窝
retroesophageal recess

心包斜窦
oblique sinu of pericardium

左心房
left atrium

右肺动脉
right pulmonary artery

右肺静脉
right pulmonary vine

右膈神经
right phrenic nerve

上腔静脉
superior vena cava

右心耳
right auricle

第 3 肋软骨
the 3th eostal cartilage

胸主动脉
thoracic aorta

胸导管
thoracic duct

食管
esophagus

左肺静脉
left pulmonary vine

左膈神经
left phrenic nerve

心包
pericardium

心包横窦
transverse sinu of pericardium

主动脉瓣
aortic valve

肺动脉瓣
pulmonary valve

图 5-17 下纵隔横断面（平第 6 胸椎体）
Lower mediastinal cross section（Flat 6th thoracic vertebra）

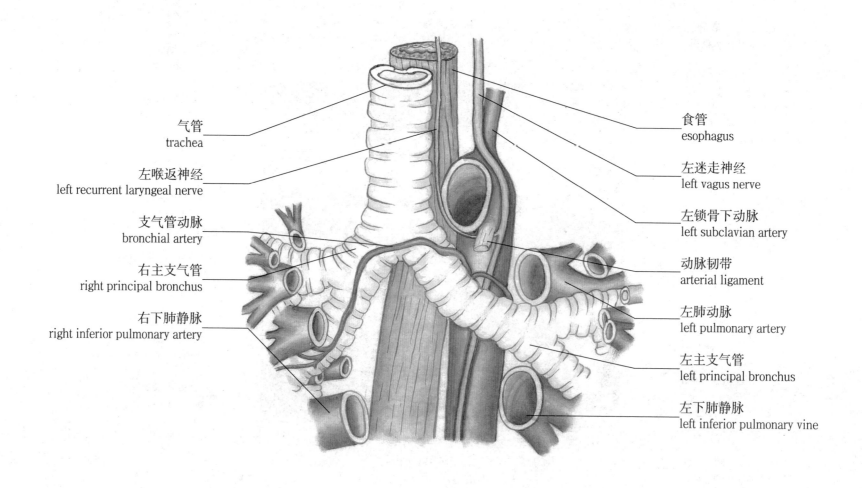

气管
trachea

左喉返神经
left recurrent laryngeal nerve

支气管动脉
bronchial artery

右主支气管
right principal bronchus

右下肺静脉
right inferior pulmonary artery

食管
esophagus

左迷走神经
left vagus nerve

左锁骨下动脉
left subclavian artery

动脉韧带
arterial ligament

左肺动脉
left pulmonary artery

左主支气管
left principal bronchus

左下肺静脉
left inferior pulmonary vine

图 5-18 气管和支气管
Trachea and bronchus

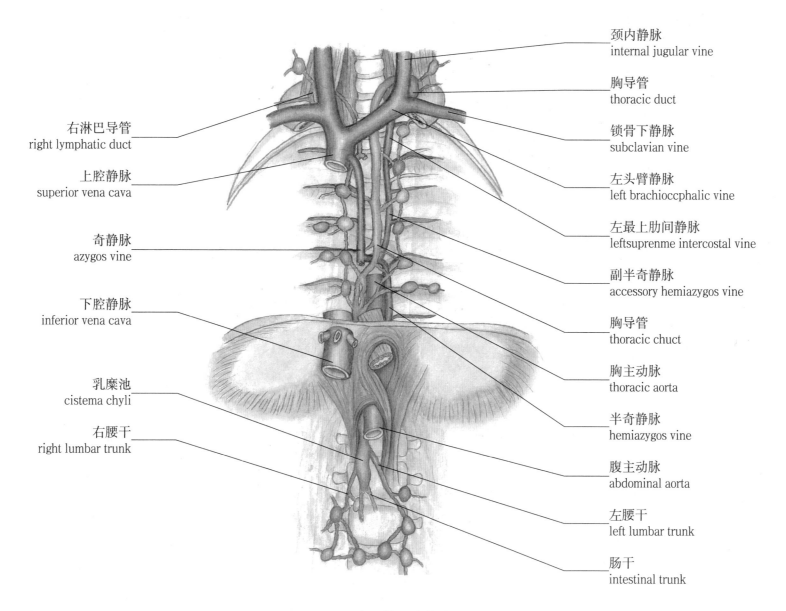

颈内静脉
internal jugular vine

胸导管
thoracic duct

锁骨下静脉
subclavian vine

左头臂静脉
left brachioccphalic vine

左最上肋间静脉
leftsuprenme intercostal vine

副半奇静脉
accessory hemiazygos vine

胸导管
thoracic chuct

胸主动脉
thoracic aorta

半奇静脉
hemiazygos vine

腹主动脉
abdominal aorta

左腰干
left lumbar trunk

肠干
intestinal trunk

右淋巴导管
right lymphatic duct

上腔静脉
superior vena cava

奇静脉
azygos vine

下腔静脉
inferior vena cava

乳糜池
cistema chyli

右腰干
right lumbar trunk

图 5-19　胸导管和奇静脉
Thoracic duct and azygos vein

腹部

第六章

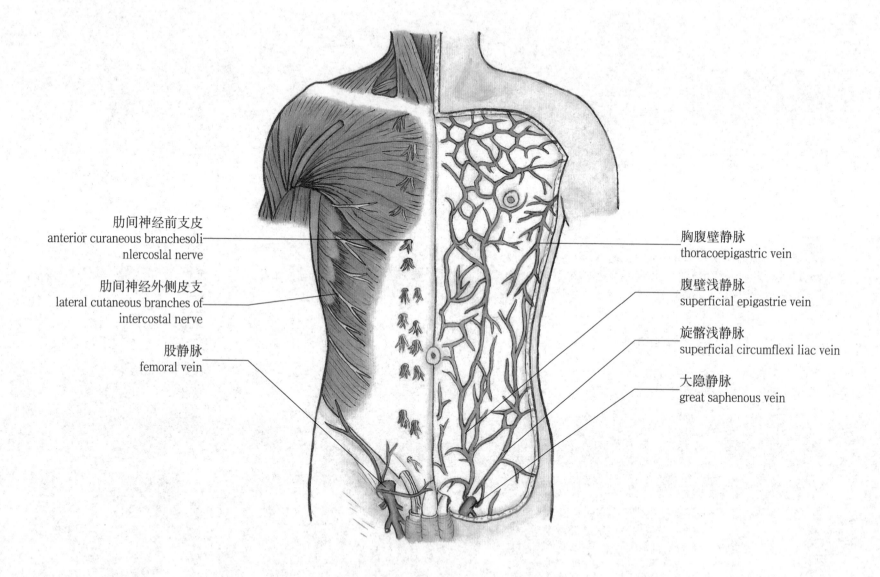

肋间神经前支皮
anterior curaneous branchesoli
nlercoslal nerve

肋间神经外侧皮支
lateral cutaneous branches of
intercostal nerve

股静脉
femoral vein

胸腹壁静脉
thoracoepigastric vein

腹壁浅静脉
superficial epigastrie vein

旋髂浅静脉
superficial circumflexi liac vein

大隐静脉
great saphenous vein

图 6-1　腹壁的皮神经和浅静脉
Cutaneous nerve and superficial artery of abdominal wall

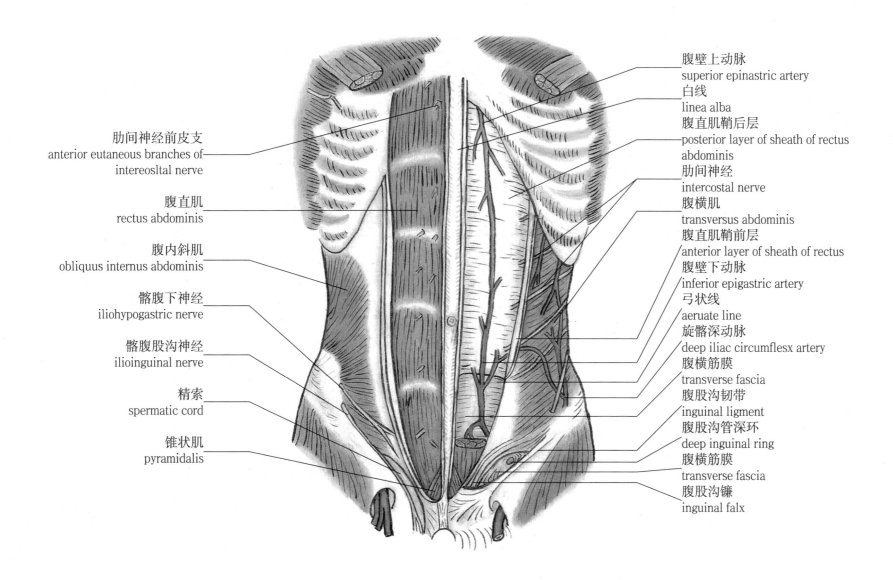

肋间神经前皮支
anterior eutaneous branches of
intereosltal nerve

腹直肌
rectus abdominis

腹内斜肌
obliquus internus abdominis

髂腹下神经
iliohypogastric nerve

髂腹股沟神经
ilioinguinal nerve

精索
spermatic cord

锥状肌
pyramidalis

腹壁上动脉
superior epinastric artery

白线
linea alba

腹直肌鞘后层
posterior layer of sheath of rectus
abdominis

肋间神经
intercostal nerve

腹横肌
transversus abdominis

腹直肌鞘前层
anterior layer of sheath of rectus

腹壁下动脉
inferior epigastric artery

弓状线
aeruate line

旋髂深动脉
deep iliac circumflesx artery

腹横筋膜
transverse fascia

腹股沟韧带
inguinal ligament

腹股沟管深环
deep inguinal ring

腹横筋膜
transverse fascia

腹股沟镰
inguinal falx

图 6-2　腹前外侧壁的肌（深层）
The muscles of the anterolateral ventral wall（deeplevel）

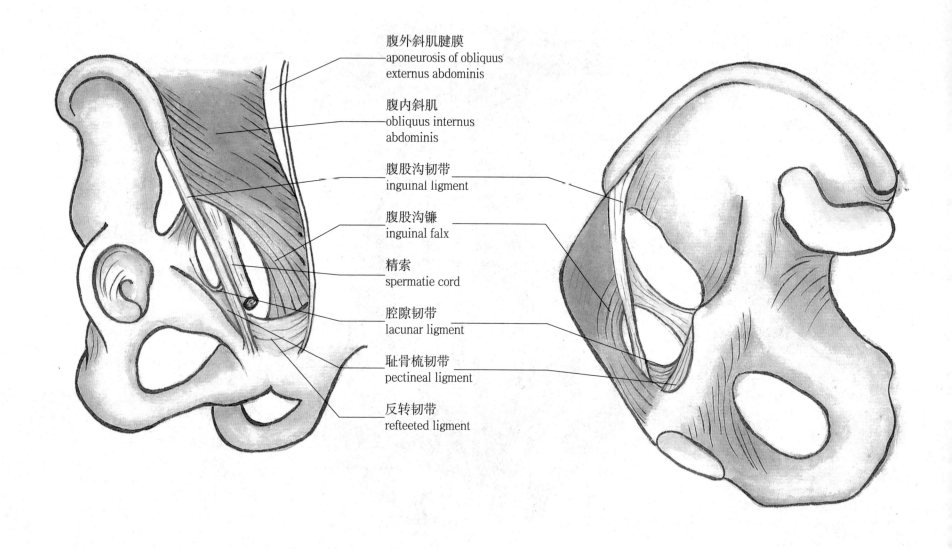

腹外斜肌腱膜
aponeurosis of obliquus
externus abdominis

腹内斜肌
obliquus internus
abdominis

腹股沟韧带
inguinal ligament

腹股沟镰
inguinal falx

精索
spermatie cord

腔隙韧带
lacunar ligment

耻骨梳韧带
pectineal ligment

反转韧带
refteeted ligment

图 6-3 腹股沟区的韧带
Ligament of inguinal region

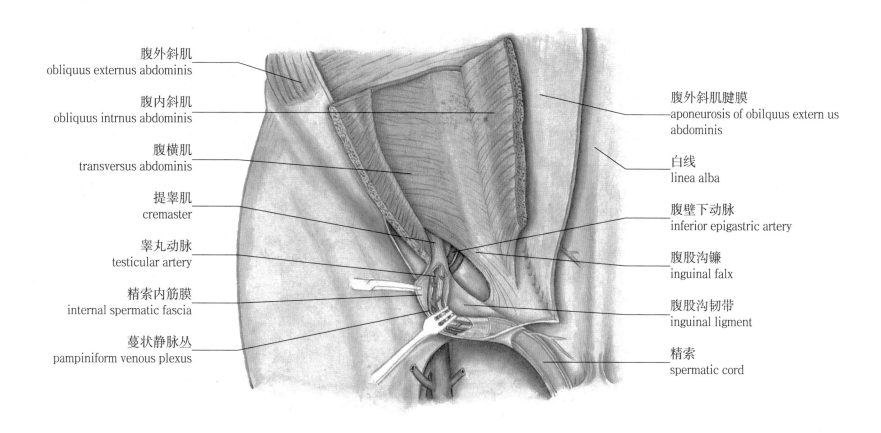

腹外斜肌
obliquus externus abdominis

腹内斜肌
obliquus intrnus abdominis

腹横肌
transversus abdominis

提睾肌
cremaster

睾丸动脉
testicular artery

精索内筋膜
internal spermatic fascia

蔓状静脉丛
pampiniform venous plexus

腹外斜肌腱膜
aponeurosis of obilquus extern us abdominis

白线
linea alba

腹壁下动脉
inferior epigastric artery

腹股沟镰
inguinal falx

腹股沟韧带
inguinal ligment

精索
spermatic cord

图 6-4 腹内斜肌、腹横肌与腹股沟镰
Internal oblique muscle,transverse abdominal muscle and sickle of groin

117

脐正中襞
median umbilical fold

脐内侧襞
medial umbilical fold

脐外侧襞
lateral umbilical fold

腹股沟外侧窝
lateral 1 inguinal fossa

腹股沟内侧窝
medial inguinal fossa

膀胱上窝
supravesical fossa

膀胱
bladder

精囊
seminal vesicle

凹间韧带
interfoveolar ligment

腹壁下动、静脉
inferior epigastrie artery and vein

腹股沟管深环
deep inguinal ring

髂外动、静脉
external iliac artery and vein

输精管
ductus deferens

前列腺
prostate

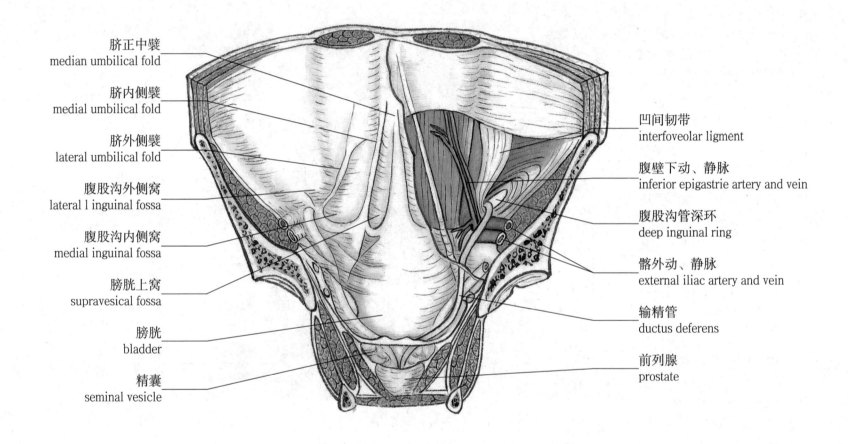

图 6-5　腹前外侧壁内面的皱襞和陷窝

Wrinkled wall and depression on the inner surface of ventral anterola teral wall

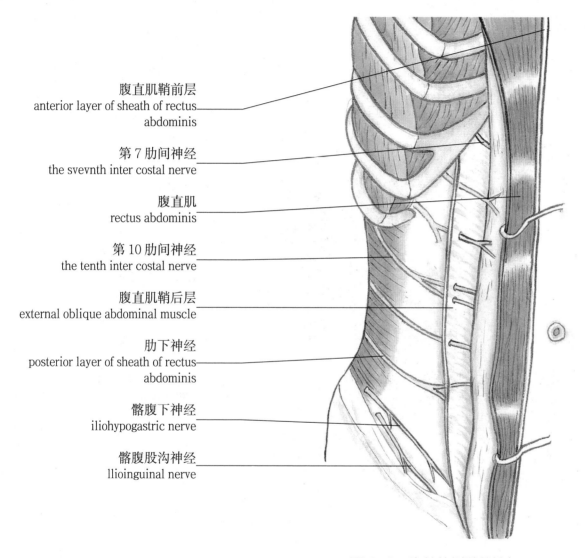

腹直肌鞘前层
anterior layer of sheath of rectus
abdominis

第 7 肋间神经
the svevnth inter costal nerve

腹直肌
rectus abdominis

第 10 肋间神经
the tenth inter costal nerve

腹直肌鞘后层
external oblique abdominal muscle

肋下神经
posterior layer of sheath of rectus
abdominis

髂腹下神经
iliohypogastric nerve

髂腹股沟神经
llioinguinal nerve

图 6-6　腹前外侧壁的神经
Nerve of ventral anterolateral wall

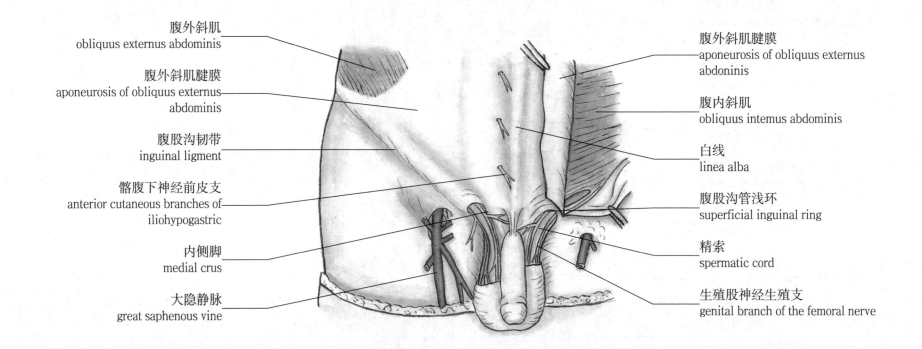

腹外斜肌
obliquus externus abdominis

腹外斜肌腱膜
aponeurosis of obliquus externus abdominis

腹股沟韧带
inguinal ligament

髂腹下神经前皮支
anterior cutaneous branches of iliohypogastric

内侧脚
medial crus

大隐静脉
great saphenous vine

腹外斜肌腱膜
aponeurosis of obliquus externus abdoninis

腹内斜肌
obliquus intemus abdominis

白线
linea alba

腹股沟管浅环
superficial inguinal ring

精索
spermatic cord

生殖股神经生殖支
genital branch of the femoral nerve

图 6-7　腹股沟管（1）
Inguinal canal（1）

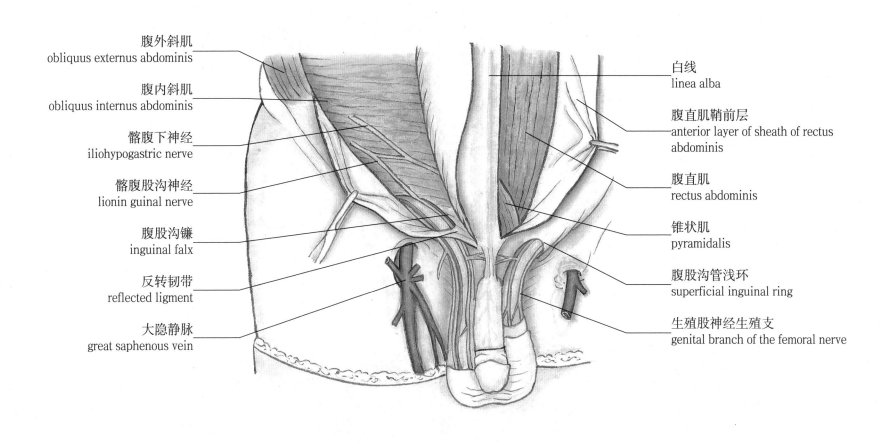

腹外斜肌
obliquus externus abdominis

腹内斜肌
obliquus internus abdominis

髂腹下神经
iliohypogastric nerve

髂腹股沟神经
lionin guinal nerve

腹股沟镰
inguinal falx

反转韧带
reflected ligment

大隐静脉
great saphenous vein

白线
linea alba

腹直肌鞘前层
anterior layer of sheath of rectus abdominis

腹直肌
rectus abdominis

锥状肌
pyramidalis

腹股沟管浅环
superficial inguinal ring

生殖股神经生殖支
genital branch of the femoral nerve

图 6-8　腹股沟管（2）
Inguinal canal（2）

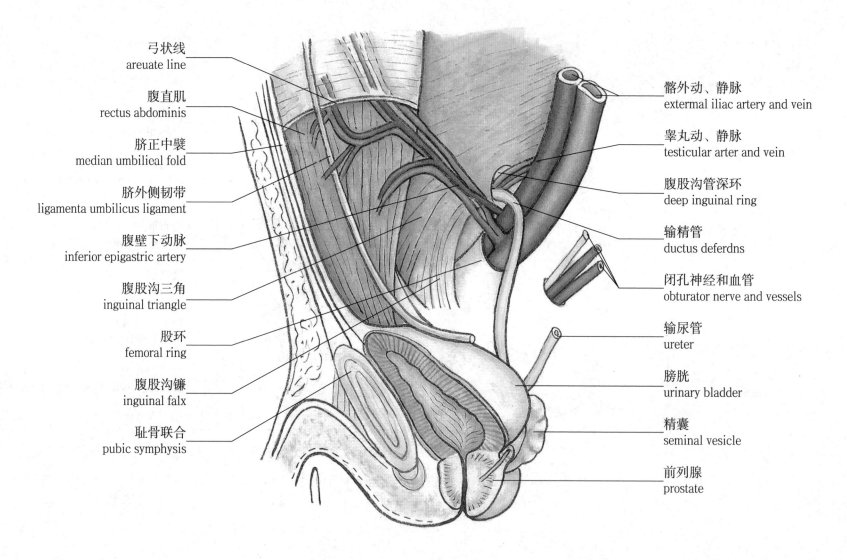

弓状线
areuate line

腹直肌
rectus abdominis

脐正中襞
median umbilical fold

脐外侧韧带
ligamenta umbilicus ligament

腹壁下动脉
inferior epigastric artery

腹股沟三角
inguinal triangle

股环
femoral ring

腹股沟镰
inguinal falx

耻骨联合
pubic symphysis

髂外动、静脉
extermal iliac artery and vein

睾丸动、静脉
testicular arter and vein

腹股沟管深环
deep inguinal ring

输精管
ductus deferdns

闭孔神经和血管
obturator nerve and vessels

输尿管
ureter

膀胱
urinary bladder

精囊
seminal vesicle

前列腺
prostate

图 6-9　腹股沟三角（内面观）
Inguinal triangle（Interior view）

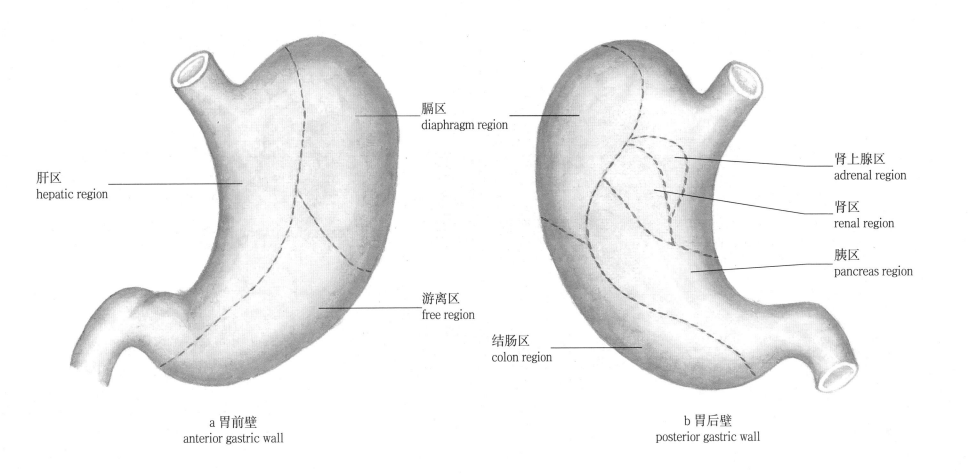

肝区
hepatic region

膈区
diaphragm region

肾上腺区
adrenal region

肾区
renal region

胰区
pancreas region

游离区
free region

结肠区
colon region

a 胃前壁
anterior gastric wall

b 胃后壁
posterior gastric wall

图 6-10 胃的毗邻
Adjacent stomach

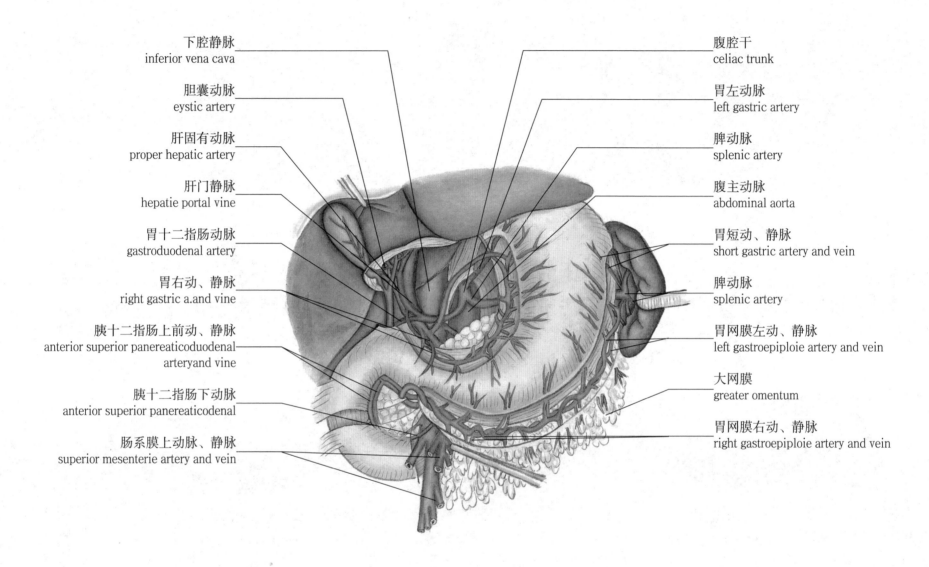

下腔静脉
inferior vena cava

胆囊动脉
eystic artery

肝固有动脉
proper hepatic artery

肝门静脉
hepatie portal vine

胃十二指肠动脉
gastroduodenal artery

胃右动、静脉
right gastric a.and vine

胰十二指肠上前动、静脉
anterior superior panereaticoduodenal
arteryand vine

胰十二指肠下动脉
anterior superior panereaticodenal

肠系膜上动脉、静脉
superior mesenterie artery and vein

腹腔干
celiac trunk

胃左动脉
left gastric artery

脾动脉
splenic artery

腹主动脉
abdominal aorta

胃短动、静脉
short gastric artery and vein

脾动脉
splenic artery

胃网膜左动、静脉
left gastroepiploie artery and vein

大网膜
greater omentum

胃网膜右动、静脉
right gastroepiploie artery and vein

图 6-11 胃的血管（前面）
Blood vessels of stomach（front）

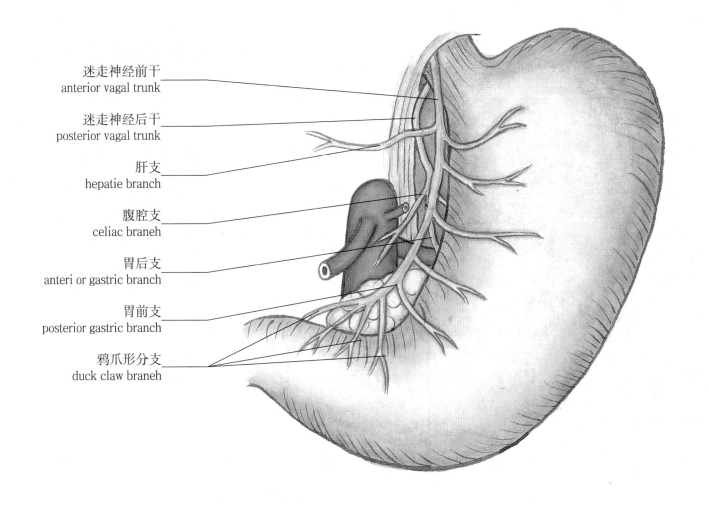

迷走神经前干
anterior vagal trunk

迷走神经后干
posterior vagal trunk

肝支
hepatie branch

腹腔支
celiac braneh

胃后支
anteri or gastric branch

胃前支
posterior gastric branch

鸦爪形分支
duck claw braneh

图 6-12　胃的迷走神经
Vagus nerve of stomach

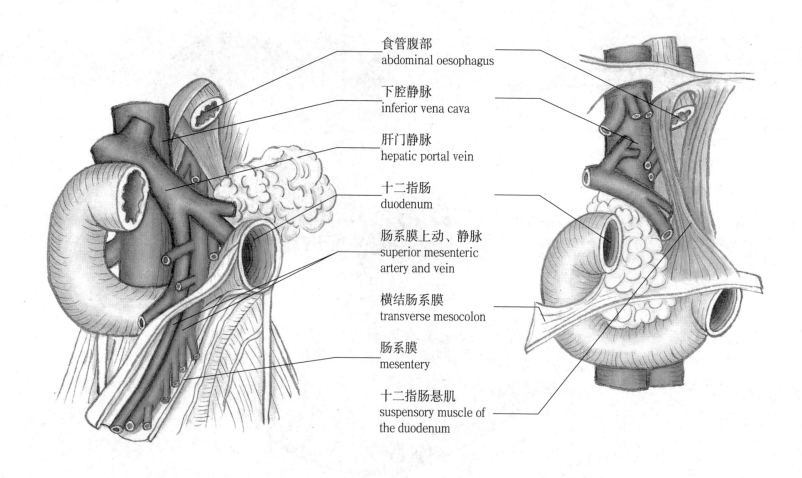

食管腹部
abdominal oesophagus

下腔静脉
inferior vena cava

肝门静脉
hepatic portal vein

十二指肠
duodenum

肠系膜上动、静脉
superior mesenteric
artery and vein

横结肠系膜
transverse mesocolon

肠系膜
mesentery

十二指肠悬肌
suspensory muscle of
the duodenum

图 6-13　十二指肠水平部的毗邻
Adjacent to the horizontal part of duodenum

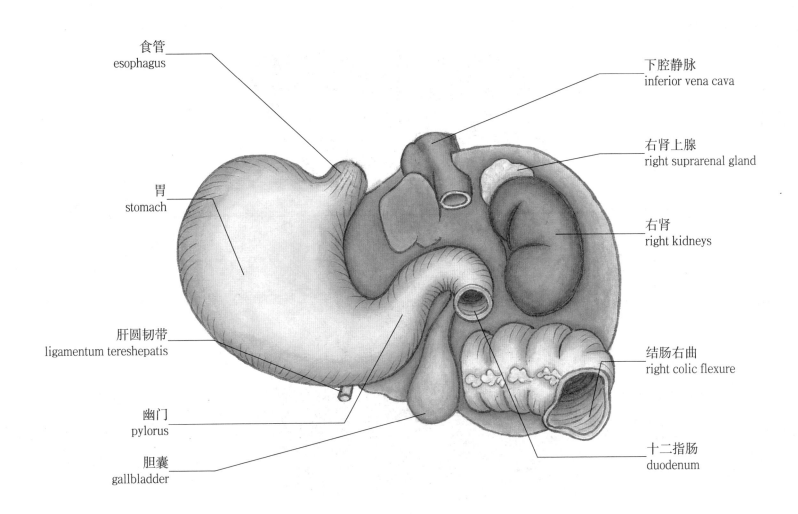

食管
esophagus

下腔静脉
inferior vena cava

胃
stomach

右肾上腺
right suprarenal gland

右肾
right kidneys

肝圆韧带
ligamentum tereshepatis

结肠右曲
right colic flexure

幽门
pylorus

十二指肠
duodenum

胆囊
gallbladder

图 6-14 肝脏面毗邻
Adjacent to liver surface

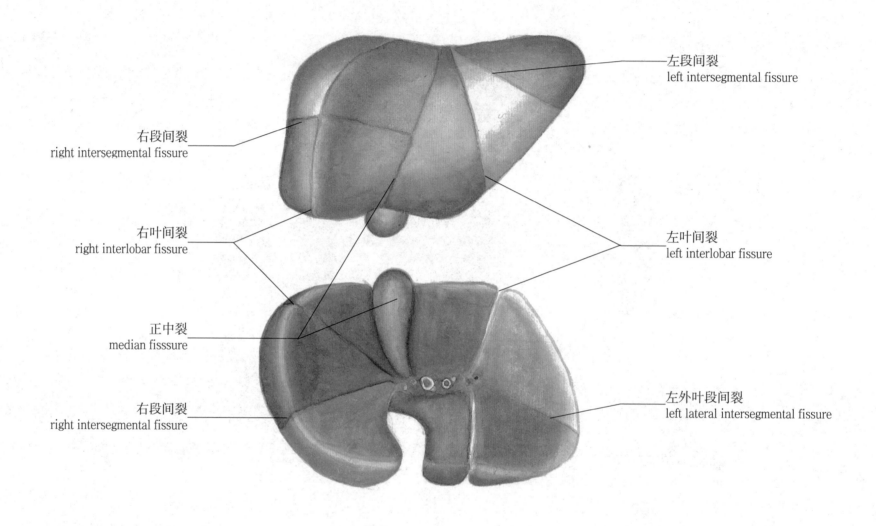

右段间裂
right intersegmental fissure

左段间裂
left intersegmental fissure

右叶间裂
right interlobar fissure

左叶间裂
left interlobar fissure

正中裂
median fisssure

右段间裂
right intersegmental fissure

左外叶段间裂
left lateral intersegmental fissure

图 6-15　肝段划分法
Liver segment division

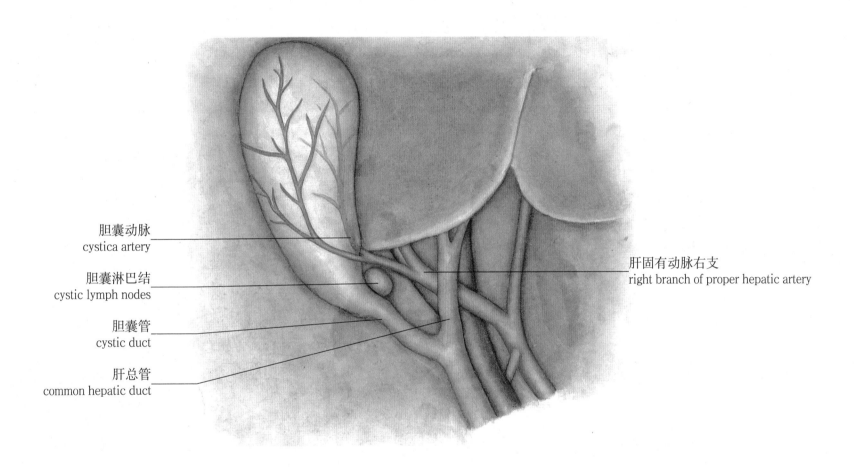

胆囊动脉
cystica artery

胆囊淋巴结
cystic lymph nodes

胆囊管
cystic duct

肝总管
common hepatic duct

肝固有动脉右支
right branch of proper hepatic artery

图 6-16　胆囊三角
Gallbladder triangle

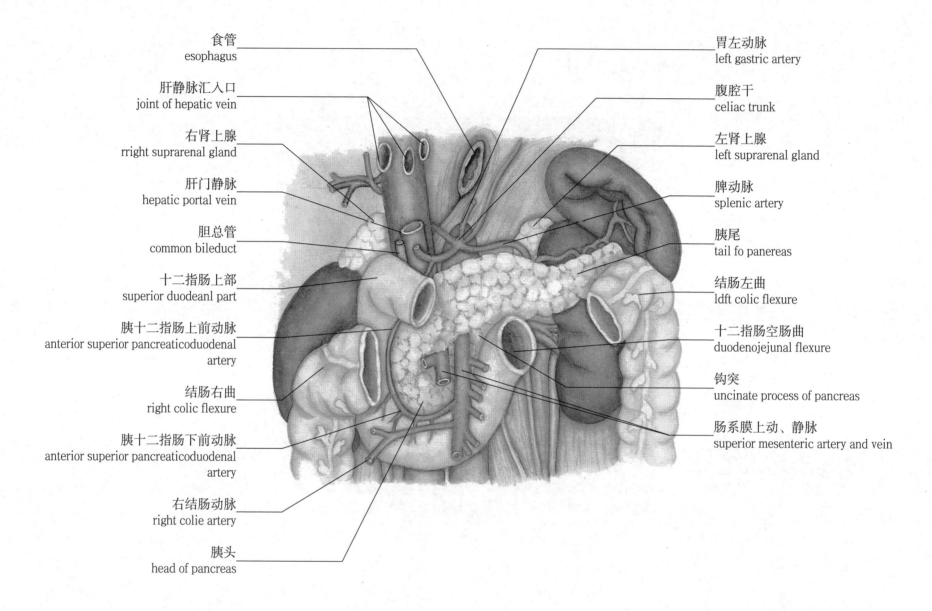

食管
esophagus

肝静脉汇入口
joint of hepatic vein

右肾上腺
rright suprarenal gland

肝门静脉
hepatic portal vein

胆总管
common bileduct

十二指肠上部
superior duodeanl part

胰十二指肠上前动脉
anterior superior pancreaticoduodenal artery

结肠右曲
right colic flexure

胰十二指肠下前动脉
anterior superior pancreaticoduodenal artery

右结肠动脉
right colie artery

胰头
head of pancreas

胃左动脉
left gastric artery

腹腔干
celiac trunk

左肾上腺
left suprarenal gland

脾动脉
splenic artery

胰尾
tail fo panereas

结肠左曲
ldft colic flexure

十二指肠空肠曲
duodenojejunal flexure

钩突
uncinate process of pancreas

肠系膜上动、静脉
superior mesenteric artery and vein

图 6-17. 胰的分部和毗邻
Division and adjacent of pancreas

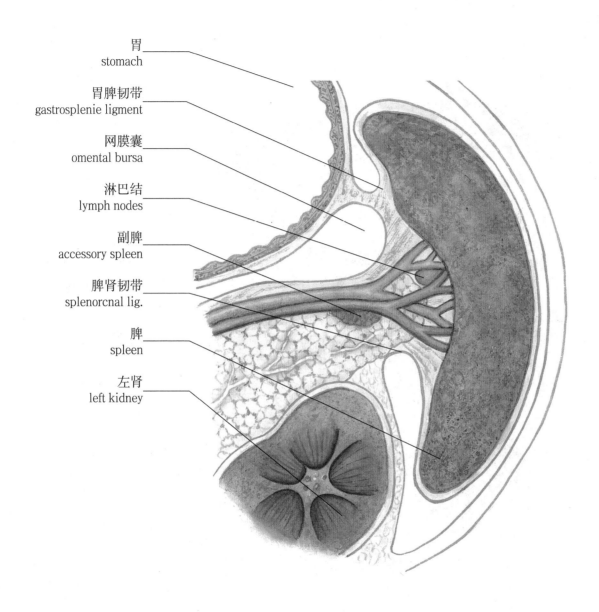

胃
stomach

胃脾韧带
gastrosplenie ligment

网膜囊
omental bursa

淋巴结
lymph nodes

副脾
accessory spleen

脾肾韧带
splenorcnal lig.

脾
spleen

左肾
left kidney

图 6-18 脾的血管和韧带
Blood vessels and ligaments of the spleen

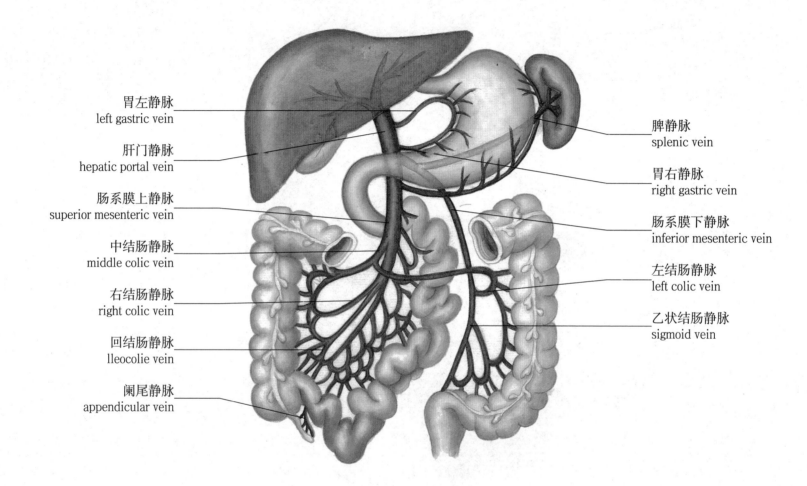

胃左静脉
left gastric vein

肝门静脉
hepatic portal vein

肠系膜上静脉
superior mesenteric vein

中结肠静脉
middle colic vein

右结肠静脉
right colic vein

回结肠静脉
lleocolie vein

阑尾静脉
appendicular vein

脾静脉
splenic vein

胃右静脉
right gastric vein

肠系膜下静脉
inferior mesenteric vein

左结肠静脉
left colic vein

乙状结肠静脉
sigmoid vein

图 6-19　肝门静脉系统
Hepatic portal vein system

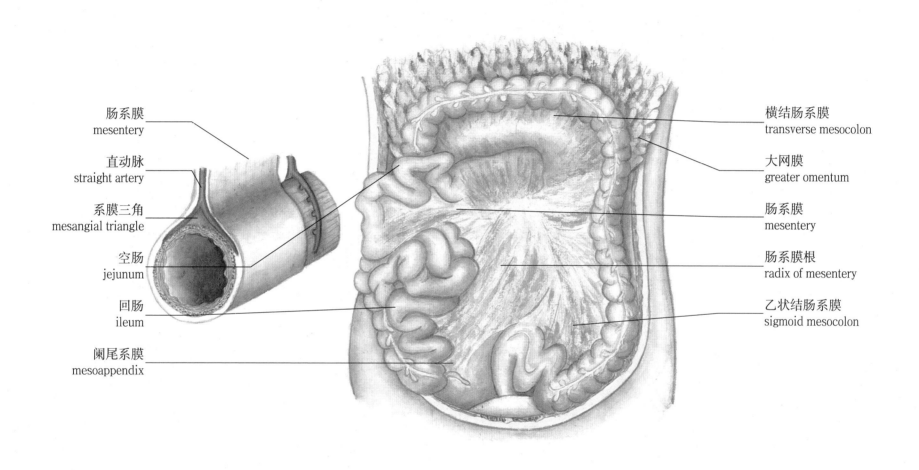

肠系膜
mesentery

直动脉
straight artery

系膜三角
mesangial triangle

空肠
jejunum

回肠
ileum

阑尾系膜
mesoappendix

横结肠系膜
transverse mesocolon

大网膜
greater omentum

肠系膜
mesentery

肠系膜根
radix of mesentery

乙状结肠系膜
sigmoid mesocolon

图 6-20 肠系膜
mesentery

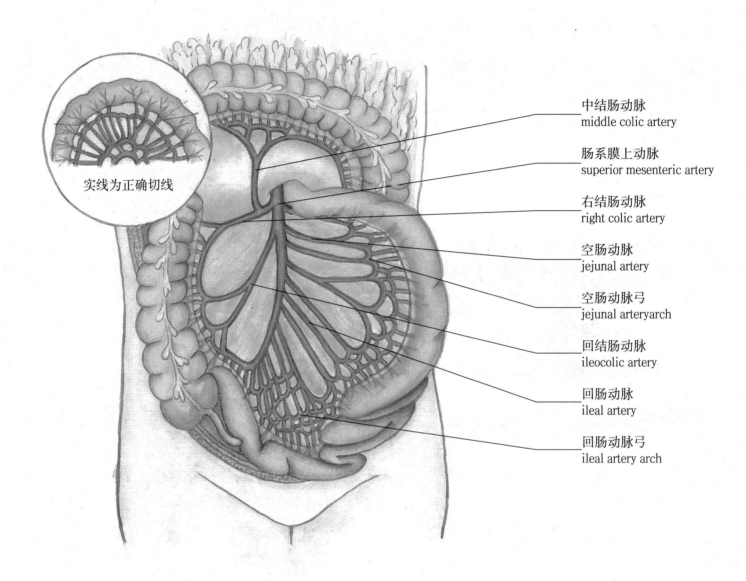

实线为正确切线

中结肠动脉
middle colic artery

肠系膜上动脉
superior mesenteric artery

右结肠动脉
right colic artery

空肠动脉
jejunal artery

空肠动脉弓
jejunal arteryarch

回结肠动脉
ileocolic artery

回肠动脉
ileal artery

回肠动脉弓
ileal artery arch

图 6-21　空、回肠的动脉
Ileal artery

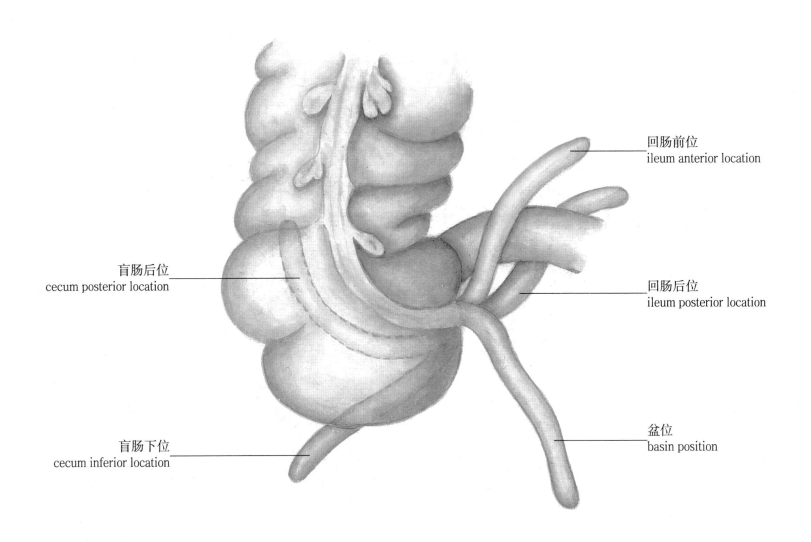

回肠前位
ileum anterior location

盲肠后位
cecum posterior location

回肠后位
ileum posterior location

盲肠下位
cecum inferior location

盆位
basin position

图 6-22 阑尾的常见位置
Commonlocation of appendix

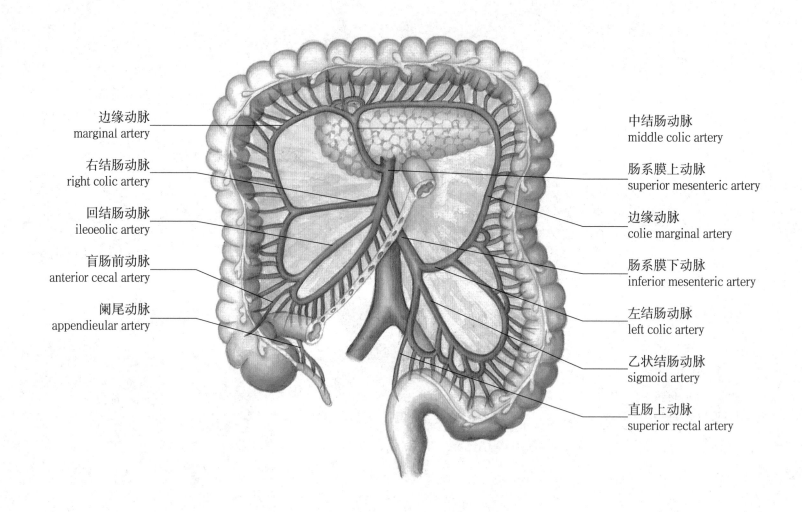

边缘动脉
marginal artery

右结肠动脉
right colic artery

回结肠动脉
ileoeolic artery

盲肠前动脉
anterior cecal artery

阑尾动脉
appendieular artery

中结肠动脉
middle colic artery

肠系膜上动脉
superior mesenteric artery

边缘动脉
colie marginal artery

肠系膜下动脉
inferior mesenteric artery

左结肠动脉
left colic artery

乙状结肠动脉
sigmoid artery

直肠上动脉
superior rectal artery

图 6-23　结肠的动脉
Arteries of colon

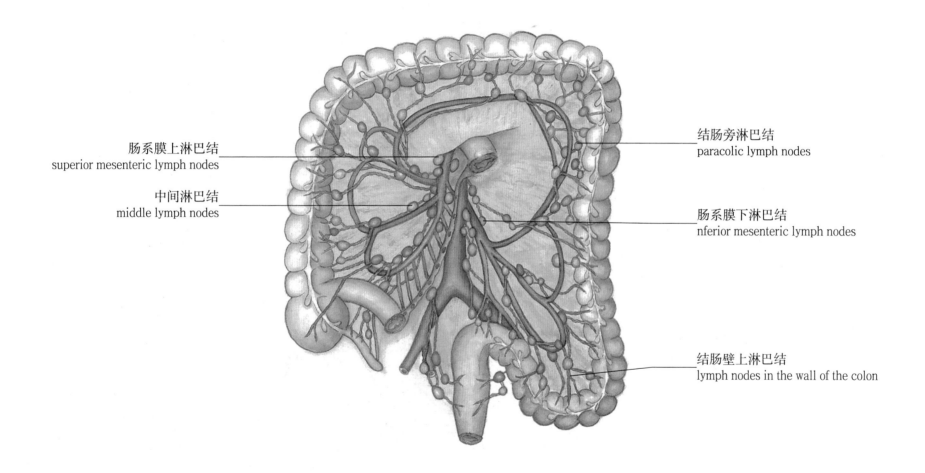

肠系膜上淋巴结
superior mesenteric lymph nodes

中间淋巴结
middle lymph nodes

结肠旁淋巴结
paracolic lymph nodes

肠系膜下淋巴结
nferior mesenteric lymph nodes

结肠壁上淋巴结
lymph nodes in the wall of the colon

图 6-24　结肠的淋巴回流
Lymphatic reflux of colon

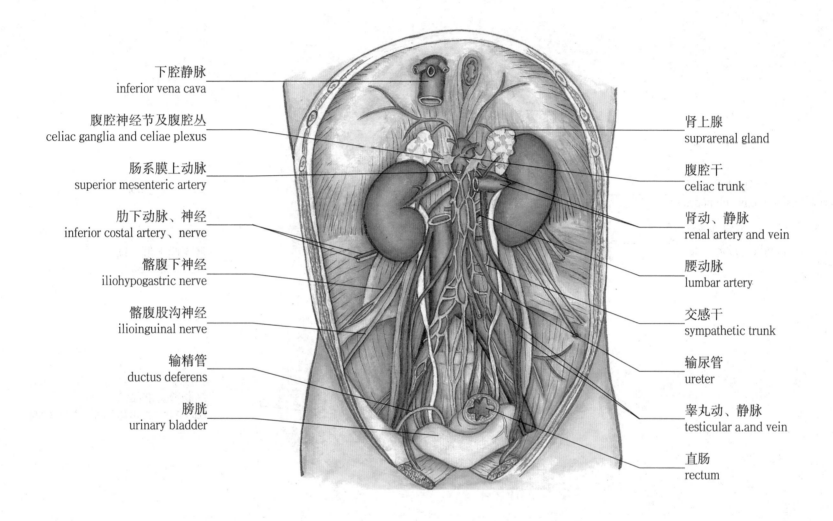

下腔静脉
inferior vena cava

腹腔神经节及腹腔丛
celiac ganglia and celiae plexus

肠系膜上动脉
superior mesenteric artery

肋下动脉、神经
inferior costal artery、nerve

髂腹下神经
iliohypogastric nerve

髂腹股沟神经
ilioinguinal nerve

输精管
ductus deferens

膀胱
urinary bladder

肾上腺
suprarenal gland

腹腔干
celiac trunk

肾动、静脉
renal artery and vein

腰动脉
lumbar artery

交感干
sympathetic trunk

输尿管
ureter

睾丸动、静脉
testicular a.and vein

直肠
rectum

图 6-25 腹膜后隙内的结构
Structure of retroperitoneal space

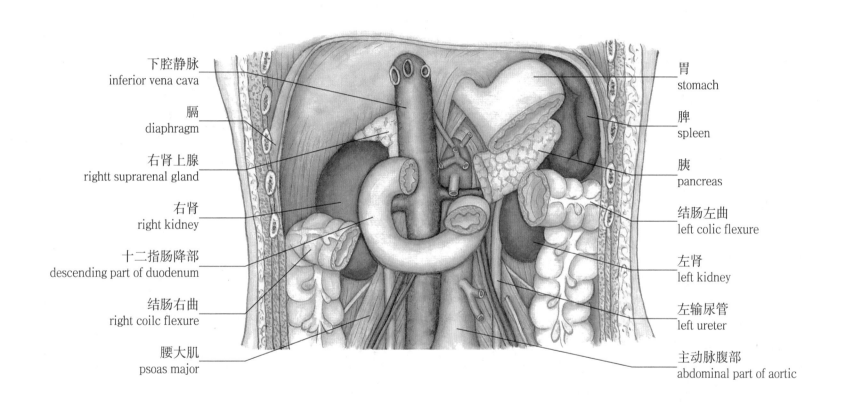

下腔静脉
inferior vena cava

膈
diaphragm

右肾上腺
rightt suprarenal gland

右肾
right kidney

十二指肠降部
descending part of duodenum

结肠右曲
right coilc flexure

腰大肌
psoas major

胃
stomach

脾
spleen

胰
pancreas

结肠左曲
left colic flexure

左肾
left kidney

左输尿管
left ureter

主动脉腹部
abdominal part of aortic

图 6-26　肾的毗邻（前面观）
Adjacent kidney（Adjacent kidney）

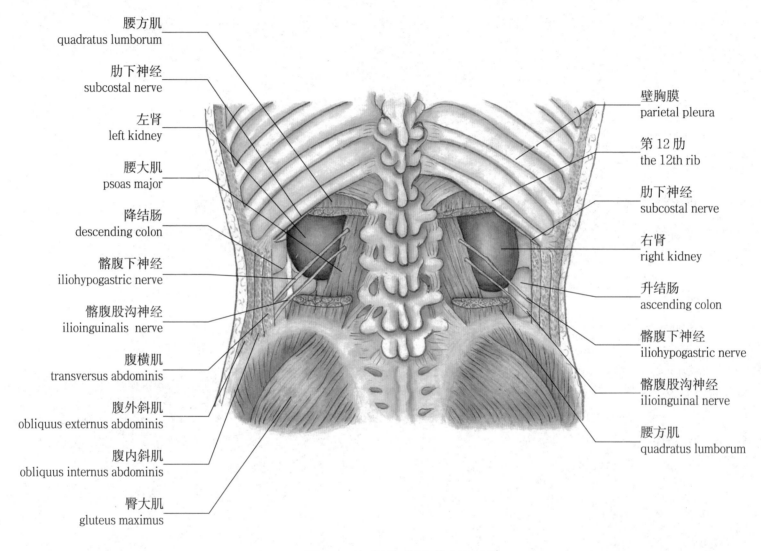

腰方肌
quadratus lumborum

肋下神经
subcostal nerve

左肾
left kidney

腰大肌
psoas major

降结肠
descending colon

髂腹下神经
iliohypogastric nerve

髂腹股沟神经
ilioinguinalis nerve

腹横肌
transversus abdominis

腹外斜肌
obliquus externus abdominis

腹内斜肌
obliquus internus abdominis

臀大肌
gluteus maximus

壁胸膜
parietal pleura

第 12 肋
the 12th rib

肋下神经
subcostal nerve

右肾
right kidney

升结肠
ascending colon

髂腹下神经
iliohypogastric nerve

髂腹股沟神经
ilioinguinal nerve

腰方肌
quadratus lumborum

图 6-27 肾的毗邻（后面观）
Adjacent kidney（Rear view）

十二指肠
duodenum

下腔静脉
inferior vena cava

腹主动脉
abdominal aorta

腹腔神经节
celiac ganglia

壁腹膜
parietal peritoneum

腹横筋膜
transverse fascia

肾前筋膜
anterior renal fascia

脂肪囊
adipose capsule of kidney

纤维囊
fibrous capsule

第 12 肋
the 12th rib

肾后筋膜
posterior renal fascia

肾旁脂体
pararenal body

腰方肌
quadratus lumborum

背阔肌
latissimus dorsi

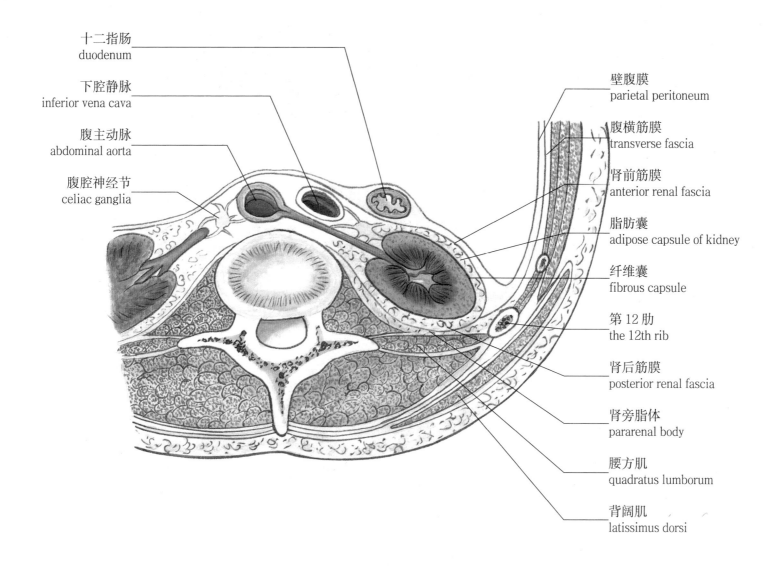

图 6-28　肾的被膜（水平切上面观）
Capsule of kidney（Horizontal cut top view）

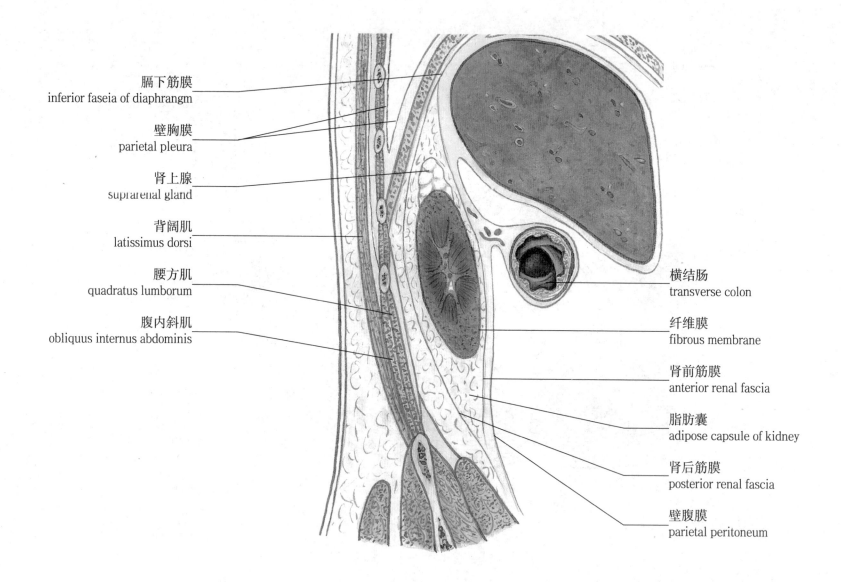

膈下筋膜
inferior faseia of diaphrangm

壁胸膜
parietal pleura

肾上腺
suprarenal gland

背阔肌
latissimus dorsi

腰方肌
quadratus lumborum

腹内斜肌
obliquus internus abdominis

横结肠
transverse colon

纤维膜
fibrous membrane

肾前筋膜
anterior renal fascia

脂肪囊
adipose capsule of kidney

肾后筋膜
posterior renal fascia

壁腹膜
parietal peritoneum

图 6-29　肾的被膜（矢状切右侧观）
Capsule of kidney（Right view of sagittal section）

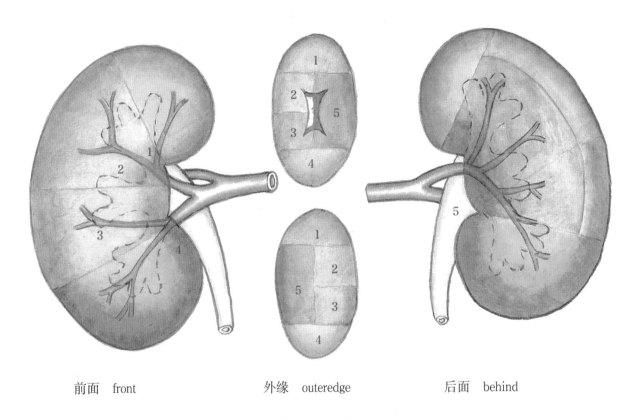

前面 front   外缘 outeredge   后面 behind

肾段动脉（右肾）
renal artery segment（right kidney）

1、上段动脉；artery of superior segment

2、上前段动脉；artery of superior anterior segment

3、下前段动脉；artery of inferior anterior segment

4、下段动脉；artery of inferior segment

5、后段动脉 :artery of posterior segment

图 6-30 右肾的肾段动脉与肾段
Renal segmental artery and renal segment of right kidney

第七章

腰背部

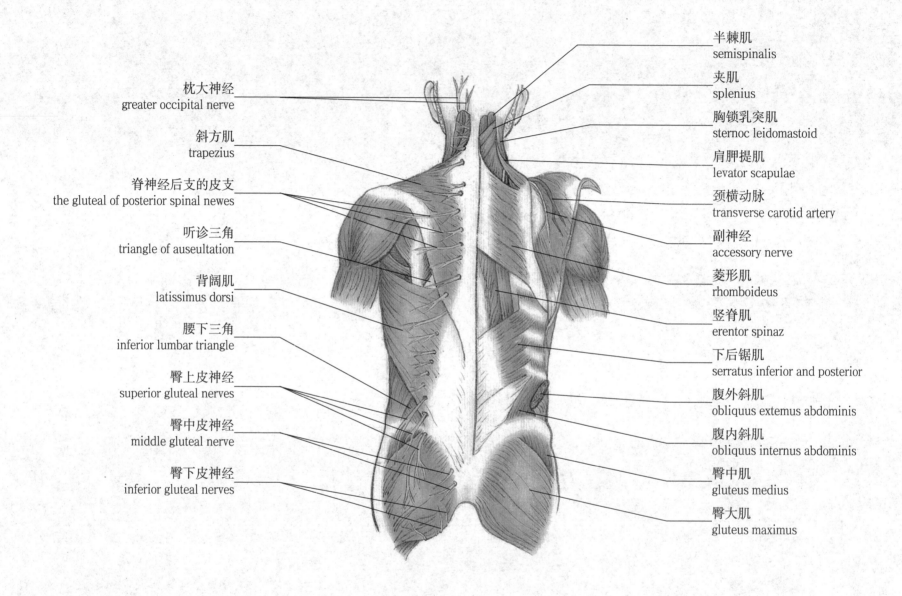

半棘肌
semispinalis

夹肌
splenius

胸锁乳突肌
sternoc leidomastoid

肩胛提肌
levator scapulae

颈横动脉
transverse carotid artery

副神经
accessory nerve

菱形肌
rhomboideus

竖脊肌
erentor spinaz

下后锯肌
serratus inferior and posterior

腹外斜肌
obliquus extemus abdominis

腹内斜肌
obliquus internus abdominis

臀中肌
gluteus medius

臀大肌
gluteus maximus

枕大神经
greater occipital nerve

斜方肌
trapezius

脊神经后支的皮支
the gluteal of posterior spinal newes

听诊三角
triangle of auseultation

背阔肌
latissimus dorsi

腰下三角
inferior lumbar triangle

臀上皮神经
superior gluteal nerves

臀中皮神经
middle gluteal nerve

臀下皮神经
inferior gluteal nerves

图 7-1　背肌及皮神经
Musckes of the back and clunial nerve

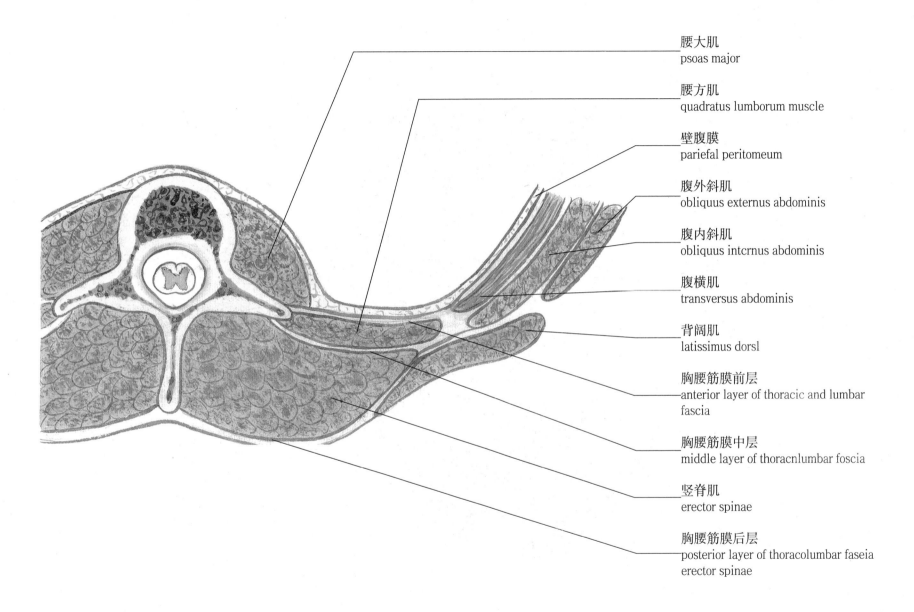

腰大肌
psoas major

腰方肌
quadratus lumborum muscle

壁腹膜
pariefal peritomeum

腹外斜肌
obliquus externus abdominis

腹内斜肌
obliquus intcrnus abdominis

腹横肌
transversus abdominis

背阔肌
latissimus dorsl

胸腰筋膜前层
anterior layer of thoracic and lumbar fascia

胸腰筋膜中层
middle layer of thoracnlumbar foscia

竖脊肌
erector spinae

胸腰筋膜后层
posterior layer of thoracolumbar faseia erector spinae

图 7-2　胸腰筋膜（水平切）
Thoraeolumbar （transverse section）

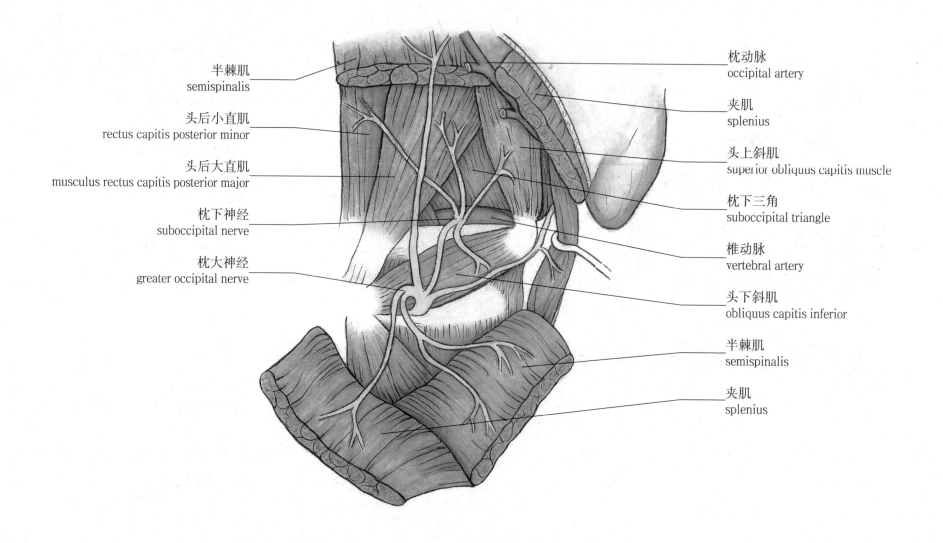

半棘肌
semispinalis

头后小直肌
rectus capitis posterior minor

头后大直肌
musculus rectus capitis posterior major

枕下神经
suboccipital nerve

枕大神经
greater occipital nerve

枕动脉
occipital artery

夹肌
splenius

头上斜肌
superior obliquus capitis muscle

枕下三角
suboccipital triangle

椎动脉
vertebral artery

头下斜肌
obliquus capitis inferior

半棘肌
semispinalis

夹肌
splenius

图 7-3　枕下三角
Suboccipital triangle

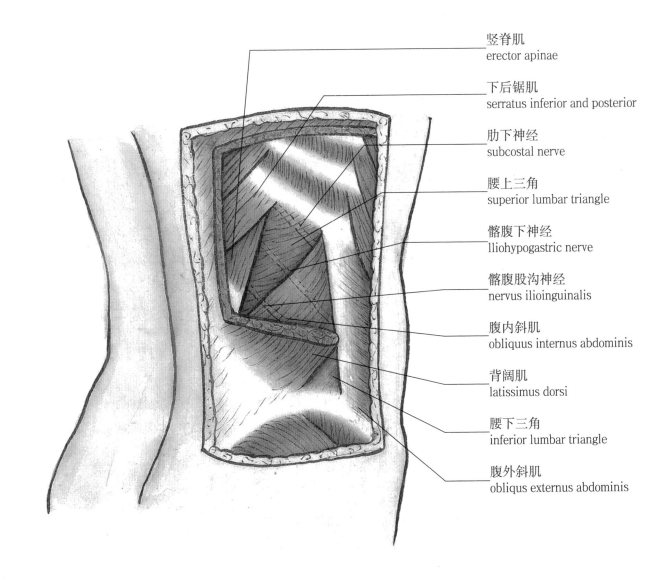

竖脊肌
erector apinae

下后锯肌
serratus inferior and posterior

肋下神经
subcostal nerve

腰上三角
superior lumbar triangle

髂腹下神经
Iliohypogastric nerve

髂腹股沟神经
nervus ilioinguinalis

腹内斜肌
obliquus internus abdominis

背阔肌
latissimus dorsi

腰下三角
inferior lumbar triangle

腹外斜肌
obliqus externus abdominis

图 7-4　腰上三角和腰下三角
Superior lumbar triangle and inferior lumbar triangle

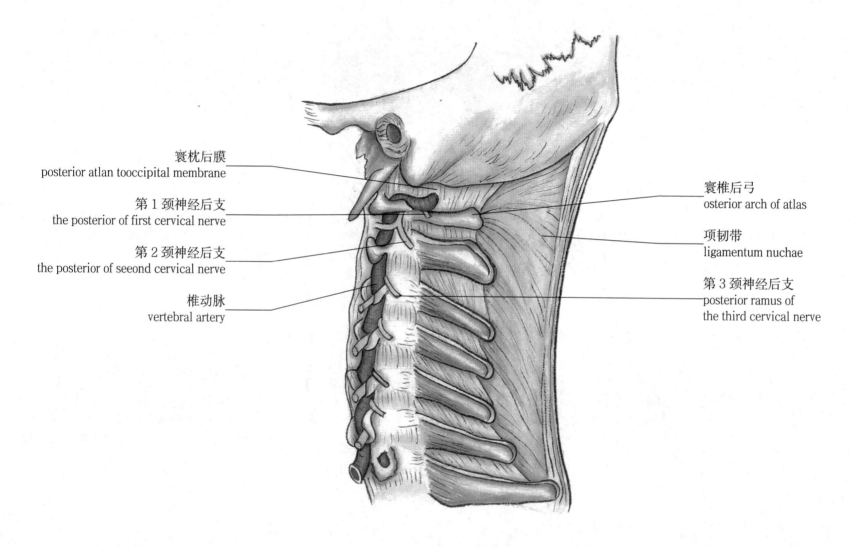

寰枕后膜
posterior atlan tooccipital membrane

第 1 颈神经后支
the posterior of first cervical nerve

第 2 颈神经后支
the posterior of seeond cervical nerve

椎动脉
vertebral artery

寰椎后弓
osterior arch of atlas

项韧带
ligamentum nuchae

第 3 颈神经后支
posterior ramus of
the third cervical nerve

图 7-5　椎动脉
Vertebral artery

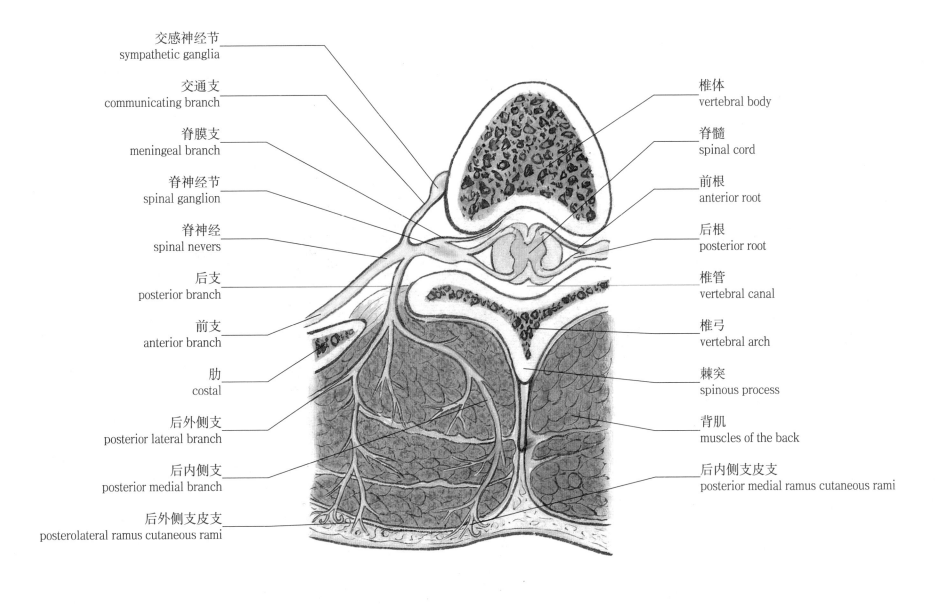

交感神经节
sympathetic ganglia

交通支
communicating branch

脊膜支
meningeal branch

脊神经节
spinal ganglion

脊神经
spinal nevers

后支
posterior branch

前支
anterior branch

肋
costal

后外侧支
posterior lateral branch

后内侧支
posterior medial branch

后外侧支皮支
posterolateral ramus cutaneous rami

椎体
vertebral body

脊髓
spinal cord

前根
anterior root

后根
posterior root

椎管
vertebral canal

椎弓
vertebral arch

棘突
spinous process

背肌
muscles of the back

后内侧支皮支
posterior medial ramus cutaneous rami

图 7-6　胸脊神经
Thoracie spinal nerves

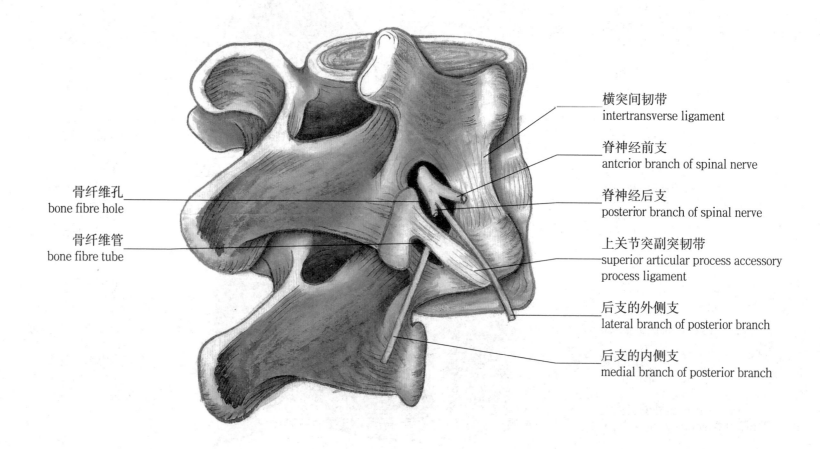

骨纤维孔
bone fibre hole

骨纤维管
bone fibre tube

横突间韧带
intertransverse ligament

脊神经前支
antcrior branch of spinal nerve

脊神经后支
posterior branch of spinal nerve

上关节突副突韧带
superior articular process accessory process ligament

后支的外侧支
lateral branch of posterior branch

后支的内侧支
medial branch of posterior branch

图 7-7　骨纤维孔和骨纤维管
Bone of fibrous foramina and canal

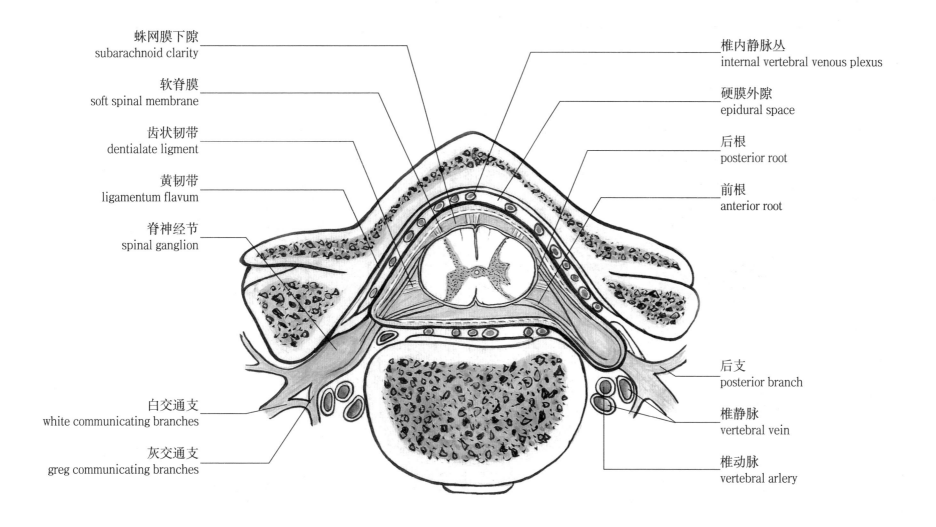

蛛网膜下隙
subarachnoid clarity

软脊膜
soft spinal membrane

齿状韧带
dentialate ligment

黄韧带
ligamentum flavum

脊神经节
spinal ganglion

白交通支
white communicating branches

灰交通支
greg communicating branches

椎内静脉丛
internal vertebral venous plexus

硬膜外隙
epidural space

后根
posterior root

前根
anterior root

后支
posterior branch

椎静脉
vertebral vein

椎动脉
vertebral arlery

图 7-8 脊髓被膜及脊膜腔隙（水平切）
Spinal cord capsule and spinal meningeal space （Horizontal section）

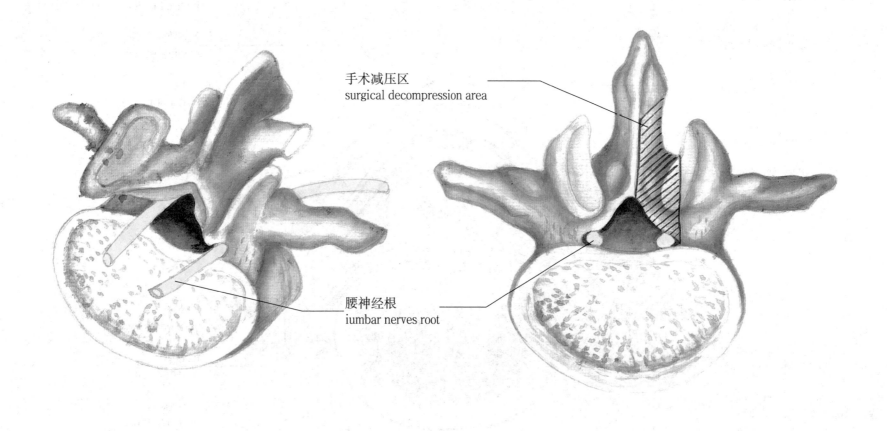

手术减压区
surgical decompression area

腰神经根
iumbar nerves root

图 7-9　椎管狭窄使神经根受压
The narrow of vertebral canal makes the nerve pressed

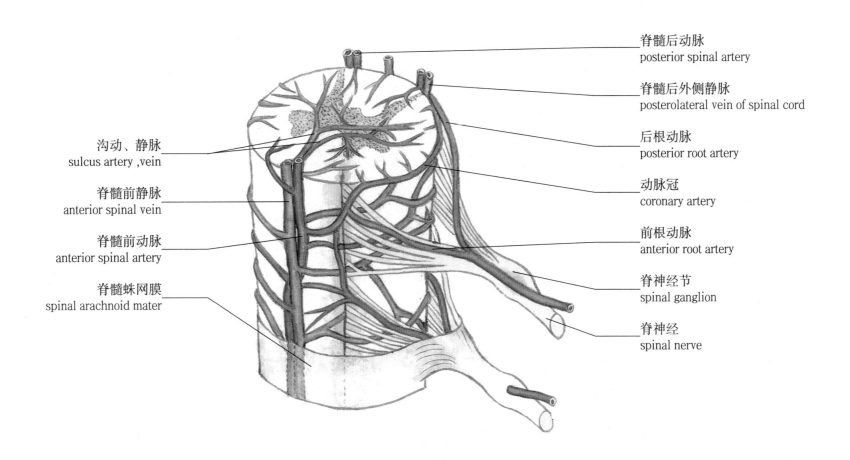

脊髓后动脉
posterior spinal artery

脊髓后外侧静脉
posterolateral vein of spinal cord

后根动脉
posterior root artery

动脉冠
coronary artery

前根动脉
anterior root artery

脊神经节
spinal ganglion

脊神经
spinal nerve

沟动、静脉
sulcus artery ,vein

脊髓前静脉
anterior spinal vein

脊髓前动脉
anterior spinal artery

脊髓蛛网膜
spinal arachnoid mater

图 7-10 脊髓的血管
The blood vessel of spinal

第八章

盆骨与会阴

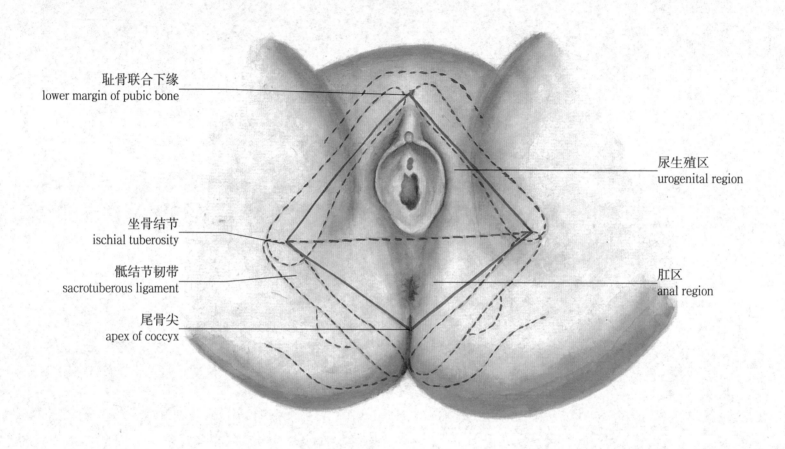

耻骨联合下缘
lower margin of pubic bone

尿生殖区
urogenital region

坐骨结节
ischial tuberosity

骶结节韧带
sacrotuberous ligament

肛区
anal region

尾骨尖
apex of coccyx

图 8-1　女性会阴分区
Subarea of female's perineum

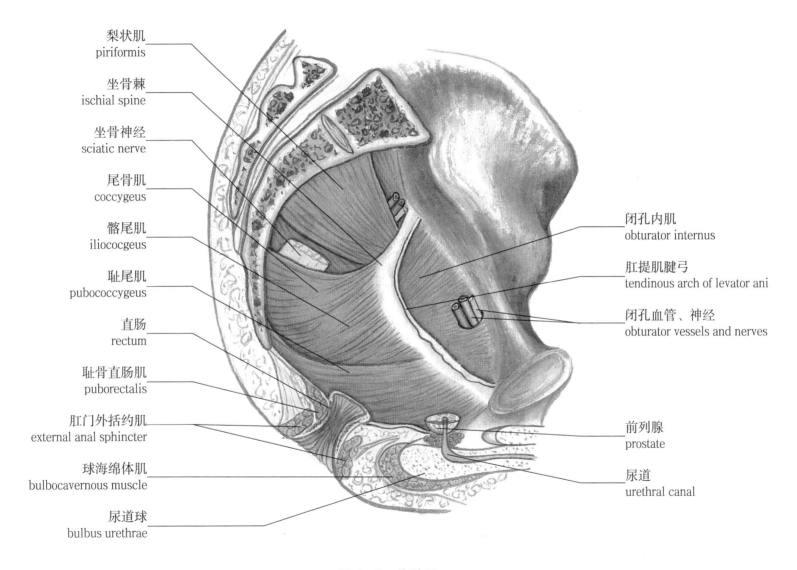

梨状肌
piriformis

坐骨棘
ischial spine

坐骨神经
sciatic nerve

尾骨肌
coccygeus

髂尾肌
iliococgeus

耻尾肌
pubococcygeus

直肠
rectum

耻骨直肠肌
puborectalis

肛门外括约肌
external anal sphincter

球海绵体肌
bulbocavernous muscle

尿道球
bulbus urethrae

闭孔内肌
obturator internus

肛提肌腱弓
tendinous arch of levator ani

闭孔血管、神经
obturator vessels and nerves

前列腺
prostate

尿道
urethral canal

图 8-2　盆壁肌
Parietal pelnic musele

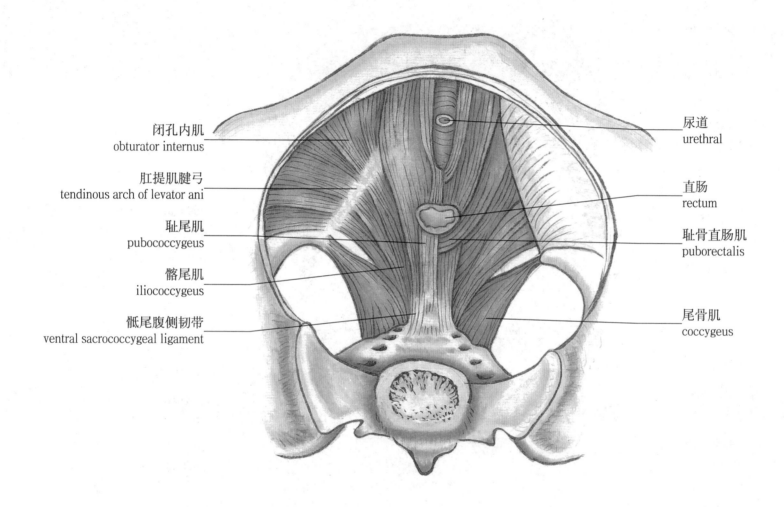

闭孔内肌
obturator internus

肛提肌腱弓
tendinous arch of levator ani

耻尾肌
pubococcygeus

髂尾肌
iliococcygeus

骶尾腹侧韧带
ventral sacrococcygeal ligament

尿道
urethral

直肠
rectum

耻骨直肠肌
puborectalis

尾骨肌
coccygeus

图 8-3 盆底肌（上面观）
Pelvic diaphragem（Inferivr aspece）

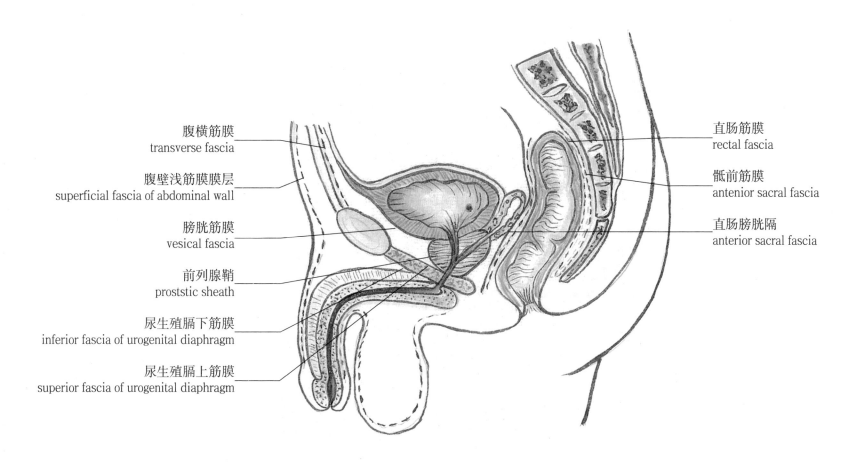

腹横筋膜
transverse fascia

腹壁浅筋膜膜层
superficial fascia of abdominal wall

膀胱筋膜
vesical fascia

前列腺鞘
proststic sheath

尿生殖膈下筋膜
inferior fascia of urogenital diaphragm

尿生殖膈上筋膜
superior fascia of urogenital diaphragm

直肠筋膜
rectal fascia

骶前筋膜
antenior sacral fascia

直肠膀胱隔
anterior sacral fascia

图 8-4　男性盆部筋膜（正中矢状面）
Median sagittal section of the male pelvic cavity foscia

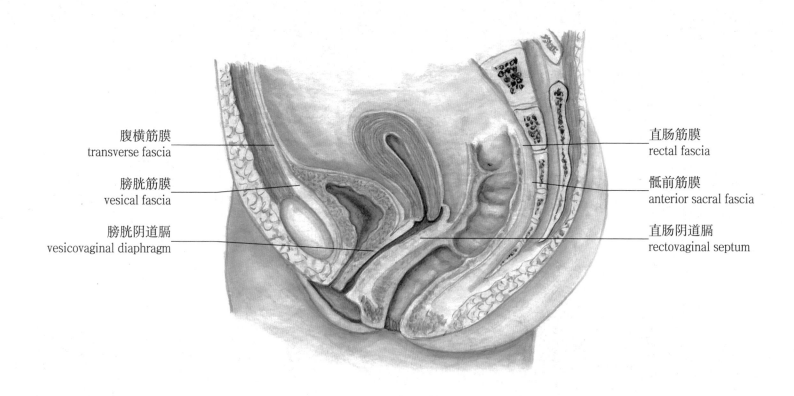

腹横筋膜
transverse fascia

膀胱筋膜
vesical fascia

膀胱阴道膈
vesicovaginal diaphragm

直肠筋膜
rectal fascia

骶前筋膜
anterior sacral fascia

直肠阴道膈
rectovaginal septum

图 8-5　女性盆部筋膜（正中矢状面）
Median sagittal aection of the female delvic part fasia

髂总动脉
common iliac artery

睾丸动脉
testicular artery

髂内动脉
internal iliac artery

髂外动脉
external iliac artery

旋髂深动脉
deep iliac circumflex artery

腹壁下动脉
inferior epigastric artery

闭孔动脉
obturator artery

闭孔神经
obturator nerve

膀胱上动脉
superior vesical artery

膀胱下动脉
inferior vesical artery

输精管
vas deferens

骶正中动脉
median sacral artery

骶外侧动脉
lateral sacral artery

臀上动脉
superior gluteal artery

骶丛
sacral plexus

臀下动脉
inferior gluteal artery

阴部内动脉
internal pudendal artery

输尿管
uretum

直肠
rectum

膀胱
urinary bladder

前列腺
ureter

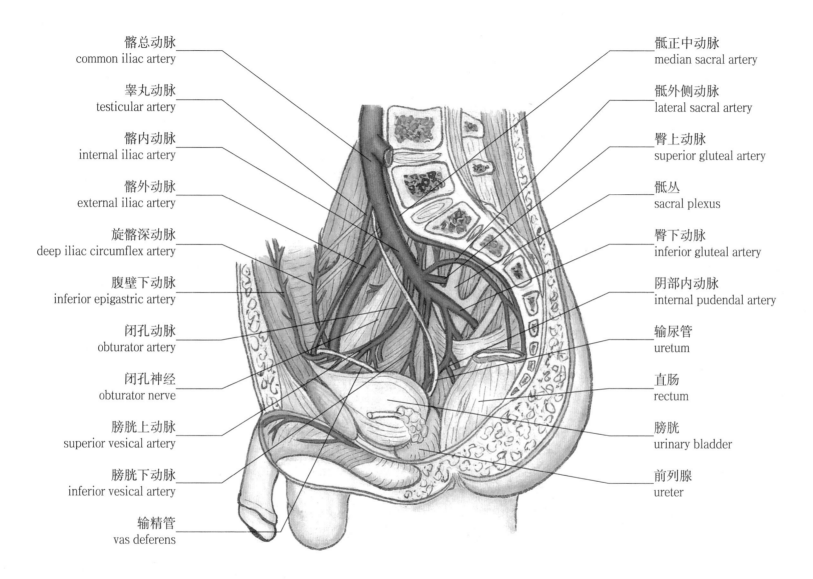

图 8-6 盆腔内的动脉
Artery of pelvic part

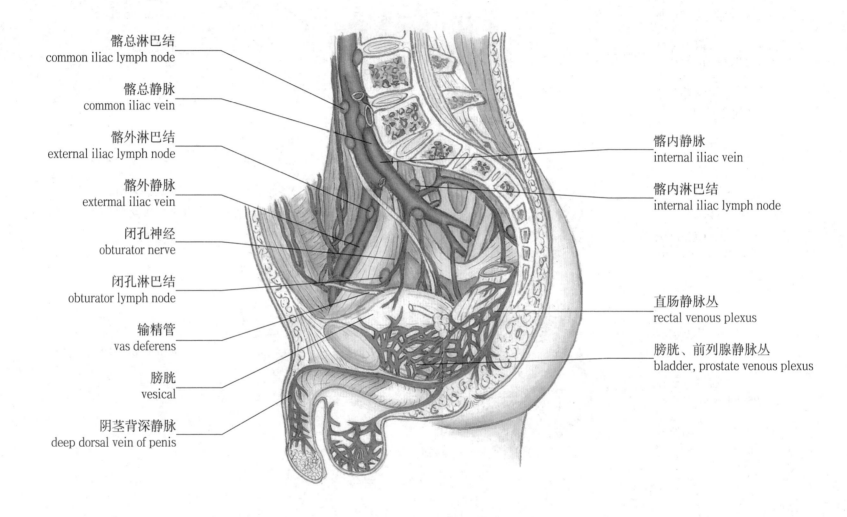

髂总淋巴结
common iliac lymph node

髂总静脉
common iliac vein

髂外淋巴结
external iliac lymph node

髂外静脉
extermal iliac vein

闭孔神经
obturator nerve

闭孔淋巴结
obturator lymph node

输精管
vas deferens

膀胱
vesical

阴茎背深静脉
deep dorsal vein of penis

髂内静脉
internal iliac vein

髂内淋巴结
internal iliac lymph node

直肠静脉丛
rectal venous plexus

膀胱、前列腺静脉丛
bladder, prostate venous plexus

图 8-7 盆部的静脉与淋巴结
Vein and lymph node of pelvic paet

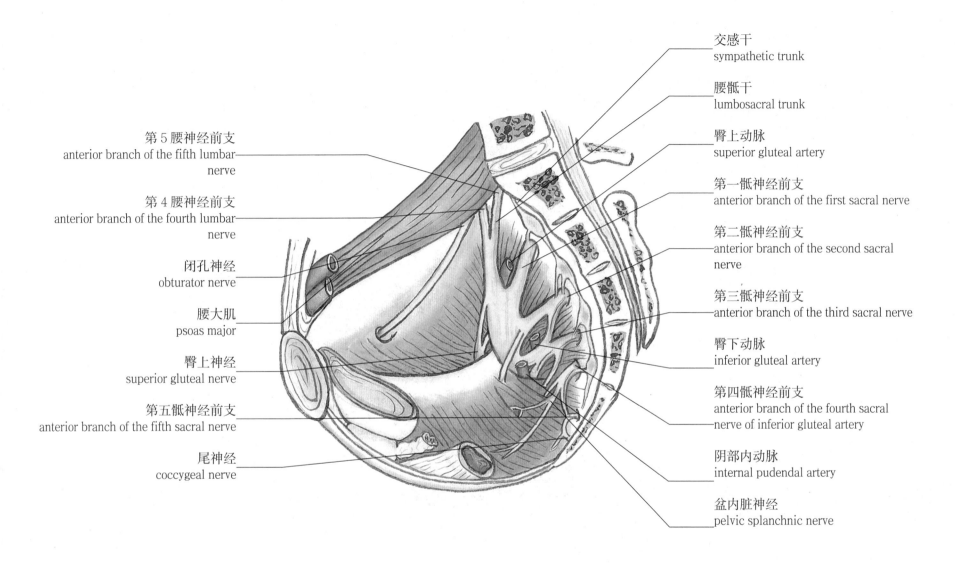

第 5 腰神经前支
anterior branch of the fifth lumbar nerve

第 4 腰神经前支
anterior branch of the fourth lumbar nerve

闭孔神经
obturator nerve

腰大肌
psoas major

臀上神经
superior gluteal nerve

第五骶神经前支
anterior branch of the fifth sacral nerve

尾神经
coccygeal nerve

交感干
sympathetic trunk

腰骶干
lumbosacral trunk

臀上动脉
superior gluteal artery

第一骶神经前支
anterior branch of the first sacral nerve

第二骶神经前支
anterior branch of the second sacral nerve

第三骶神经前支
anterior branch of the third sacral nerve

臀下动脉
inferior gluteal artery

第四骶神经前支
anterior branch of the fourth sacral nerve of inferior gluteal artery

阴部内动脉
internal pudendal artery

盆内脏神经
pelvic splanchnic nerve

图 8-8　骶丛和尾丛
Sacral plexus and coccygeal plexus

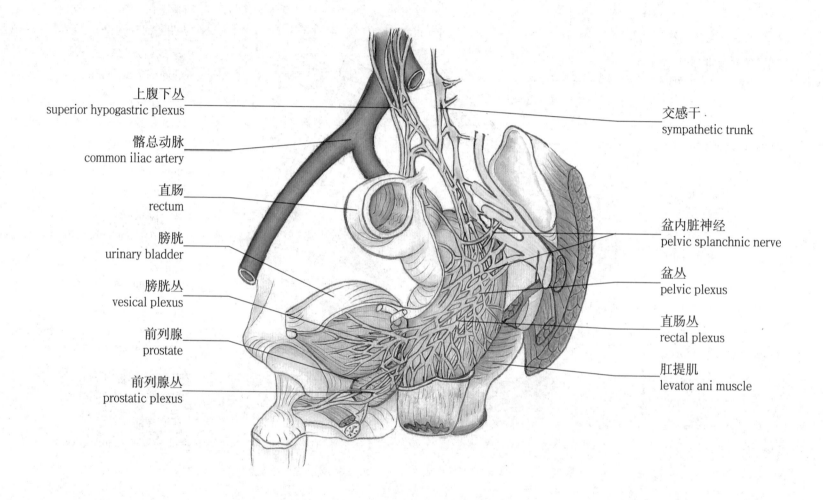

上腹下丛
superior hypogastric plexus

髂总动脉
common iliac artery

直肠
rectum

膀胱
urinary bladder

膀胱丛
vesical plexus

前列腺
prostate

前列腺丛
prostatic plexus

交感干
sympathetic trunk

盆内脏神经
pelvic splanchnic nerve

盆丛
pelvic plexus

直肠丛
rectal plexus

肛提肌
levator ani muscle

图 8-9　盆部的内脏神结
Visceral nerve of pelvic part

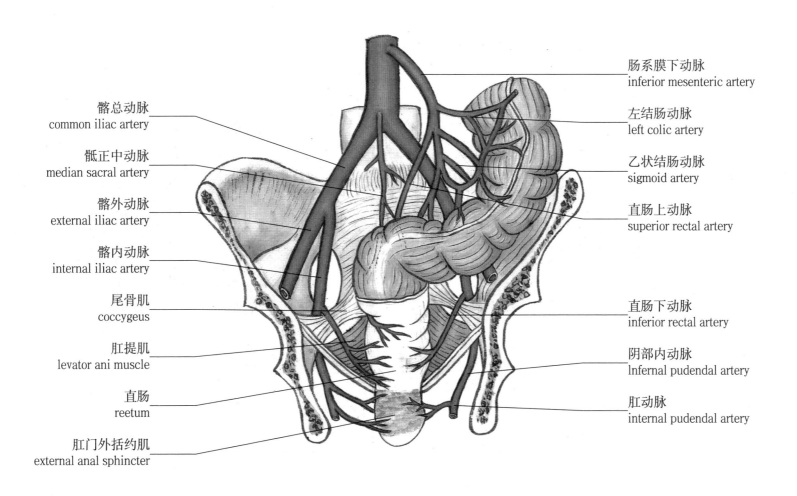

肠系膜下动脉
inferior mesenteric artery

左结肠动脉
left colic artery

乙状结肠动脉
sigmoid artery

直肠上动脉
superior rectal artery

直肠下动脉
inferior rectal artery

阴部内动脉
lnfernal pudendal artery

肛动脉
internal pudendal artery

髂总动脉
common iliac artery

骶正中动脉
median sacral artery

髂外动脉
external iliac artery

髂内动脉
internal iliac artery

尾骨肌
coccygeus

肛提肌
levator ani muscle

直肠
reetum

肛门外括约肌
external anal sphincter

图 8-10　直肠和肛管的动脉（后面观）
The artery of retum and anal canal（posterior view）

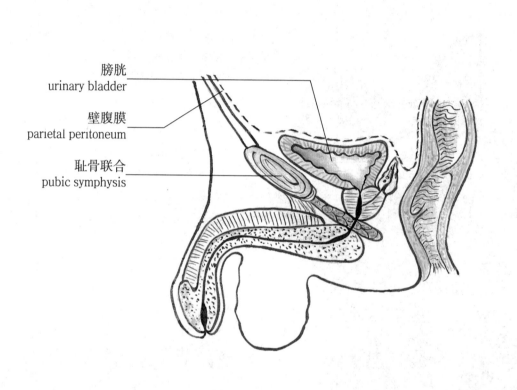

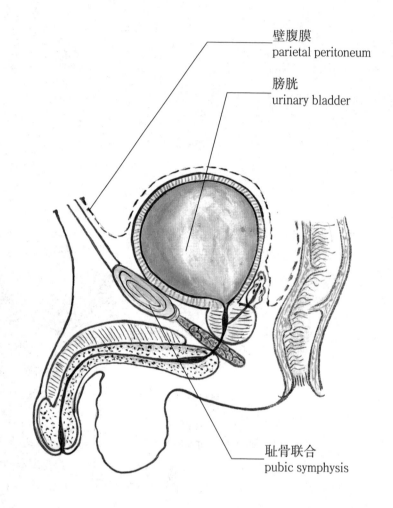

膀胱
urinary bladder

壁腹膜
parietal peritoneum

耻骨联合
pubic symphysis

壁腹膜
parietal peritoneum

膀胱
urinary bladder

耻骨联合
pubic symphysis

图 8-11　膀胱的形态与位置变化

Morphological and positional changes of bladder

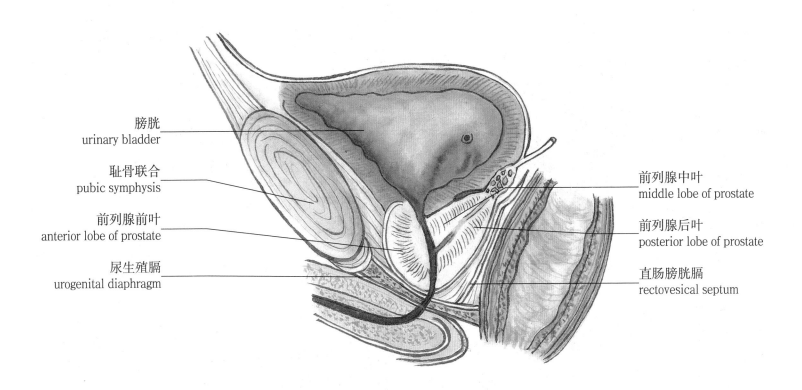

膀胱
urinary bladder

耻骨联合
pubic symphysis

前列腺前叶
anterior lobe of prostate

尿生殖膈
urogenital diaphragm

前列腺中叶
middle lobe of prostate

前列腺后叶
posterior lobe of prostate

直肠膀胱膈
rectovesical septum

图 8-12　前列腺的位置
The postion of prostate

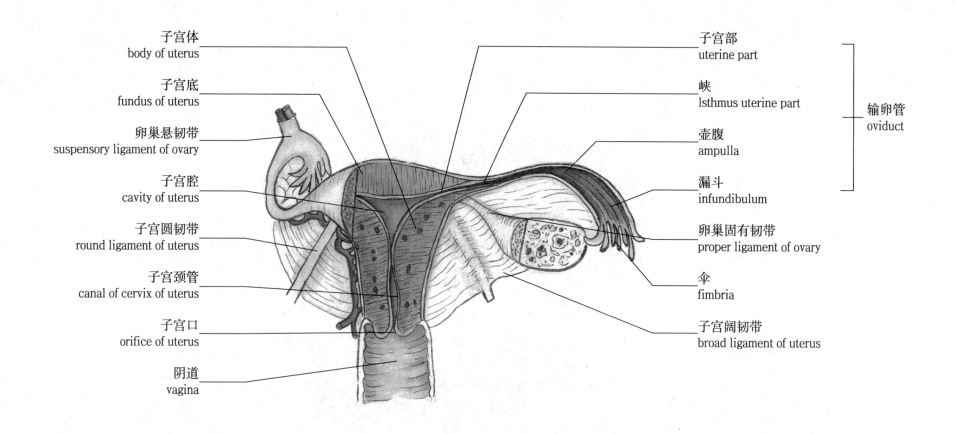

子宫体
body of uterus

子宫底
fundus of uterus

卵巢悬韧带
suspensory ligament of ovary

子宫腔
cavity of uterus

子宫圆韧带
round ligament of uterus

子宫颈管
canal of cervix of uterus

子宫口
orifice of uterus

阴道
vagina

子宫部
uterine part

峡
lsthmus uterine part

壶腹
ampulla

漏斗
infundibulum

卵巢固有韧带
proper ligament of ovary

伞
fimbria

子宫阔韧带
broad ligament of uterus

输卵管
oviduct

图 8-13 子宫的韧带
The uterus ligament

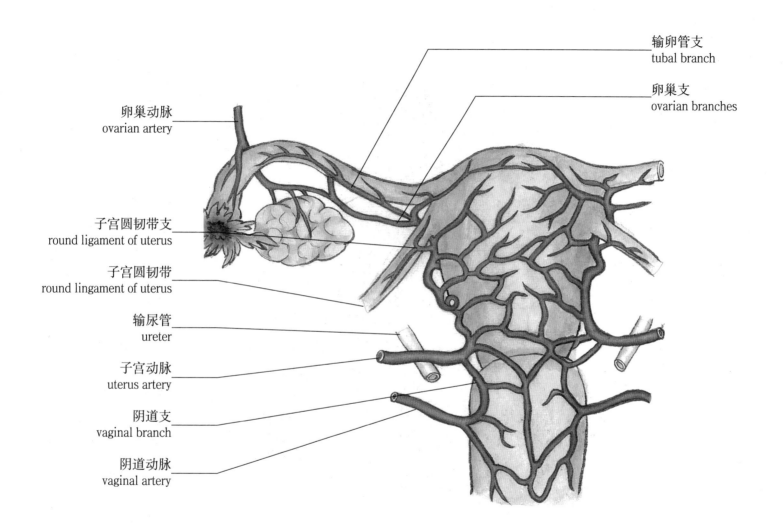

输卵管支
tubal branch

卵巢支
ovarian branches

卵巢动脉
ovarian artery

子宫圆韧带支
round ligament of uterus

子宫圆韧带
round lingament of uterus

输尿管
ureter

子宫动脉
uterus artery

阴道支
vaginal branch

阴道动脉
vaginal artery

图 8-14　女性内生殖器的动脉
The artery of female s genital organ

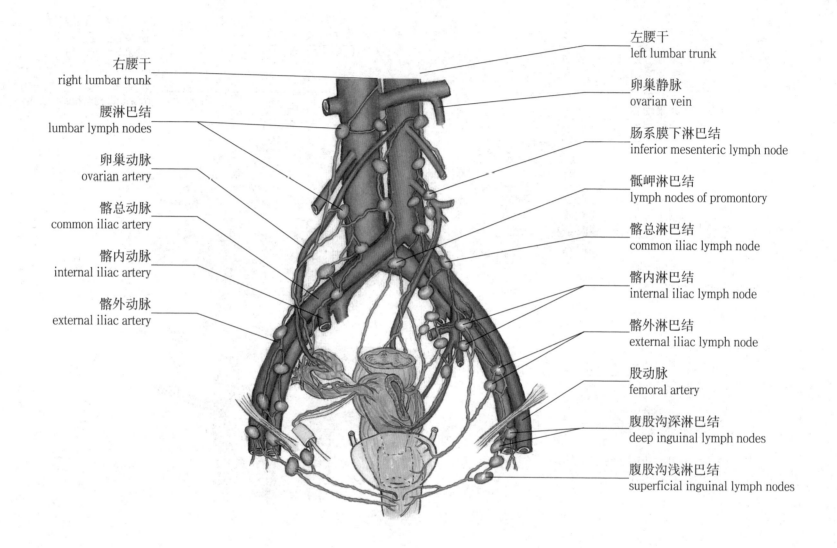

右腰干
right lumbar trunk

腰淋巴结
lumbar lymph nodes

卵巢动脉
ovarian artery

髂总动脉
common iliac artery

髂内动脉
internal iliac artery

髂外动脉
external iliac artery

左腰干
left lumbar trunk

卵巢静脉
ovarian vein

肠系膜下淋巴结
inferior mesenteric lymph node

骶岬淋巴结
lymph nodes of promontory

髂总淋巴结
common iliac lymph node

髂内淋巴结
internal iliac lymph node

髂外淋巴结
external iliac lymph node

股动脉
femoral artery

腹股沟深淋巴结
deep inguinal lymph nodes

腹股沟浅淋巴结
superficial inguinal lymph nodes

图 8-15　女性生殖器的淋巴引流
The lymph node of female's organ

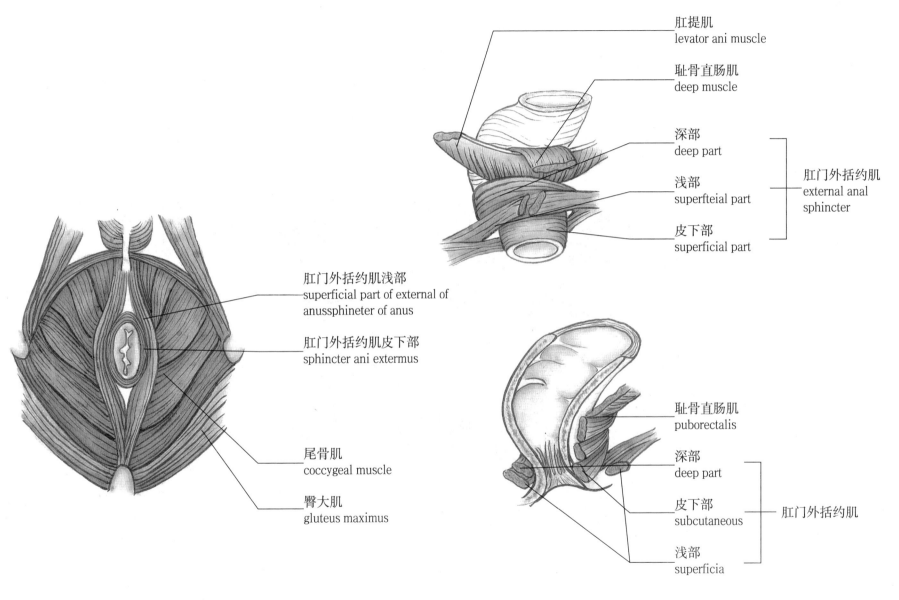

肛提肌
levator ani muscle

耻骨直肠肌
deep muscle

深部
deep part

浅部
superfteial part

皮下部
superficial part

肛门外括约肌
external anal sphincter

肛门外括约肌浅部
superficial part of external of
anussphineter of anus

肛门外括约肌皮下部
sphincter ani extermus

尾骨肌
coccygeal muscle

臀大肌
gluteus maximus

耻骨直肠肌
puborectalis

深部
deep part

皮下部
subcutaneous

浅部
superficia

肛门外括约肌

图 8-16 肛门括约肌
Anal aphincter

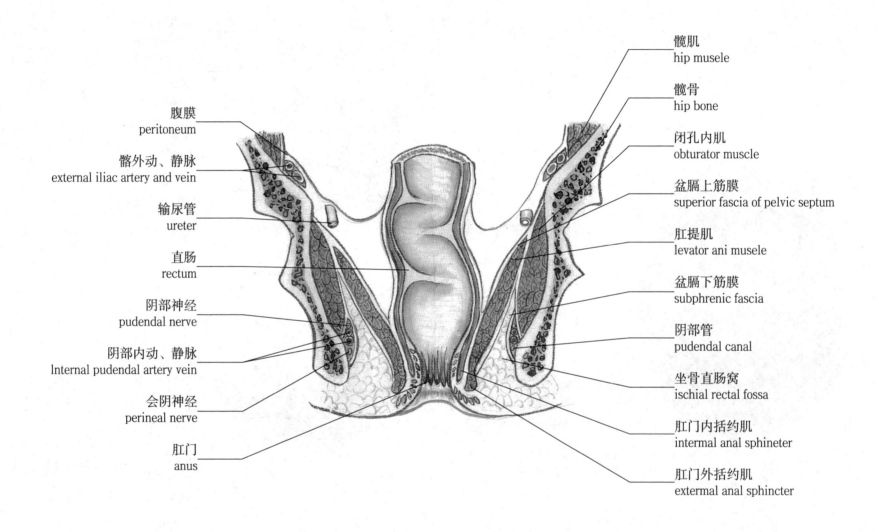

髋肌
hip musele

髋骨
hip bone

闭孔内肌
obturator muscle

盆膈上筋膜
superior fascia of pelvic septum

肛提肌
levator ani musele

盆膈下筋膜
subphrenic fascia

阴部管
pudendal canal

坐骨直肠窝
ischial rectal fossa

肛门内括约肌
intermal anal shineter

肛门外括约肌
extermal anal sphincter

腹膜
peritoneum

髂外动、静脉
external iliac artery and vein

输尿管
ureter

直肠
rectum

阴部神经
pudendal nerve

阴部内动、静脉
lnternal pudendal artery vein

会阴神经
perineal nerve

肛门
anus

图 8-17 坐骨直肠窝
Ischiorectal fossa

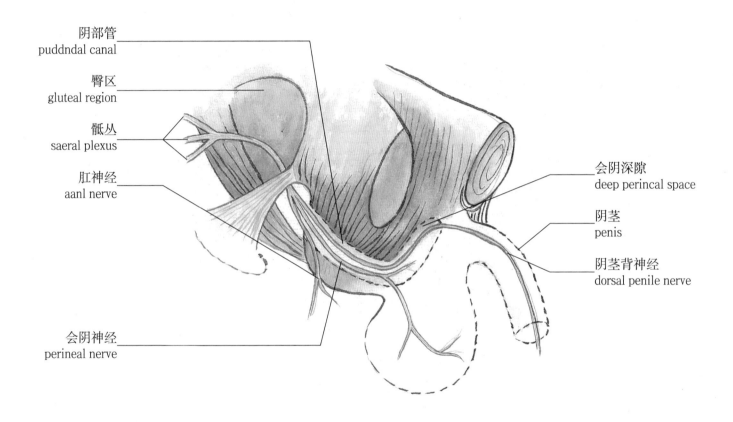

阴部管
puddndal canal

臀区
gluteal region

骶丛
saeral plexus

肛神经
aanl nerve

会阴神经
perineal nerve

会阴深隙
deep perincal space

阴茎
penis

阴茎背神经
dorsal penile nerve

图 8-18　阴部神经的行程和分支
Pan and branch of the pudendal nerve

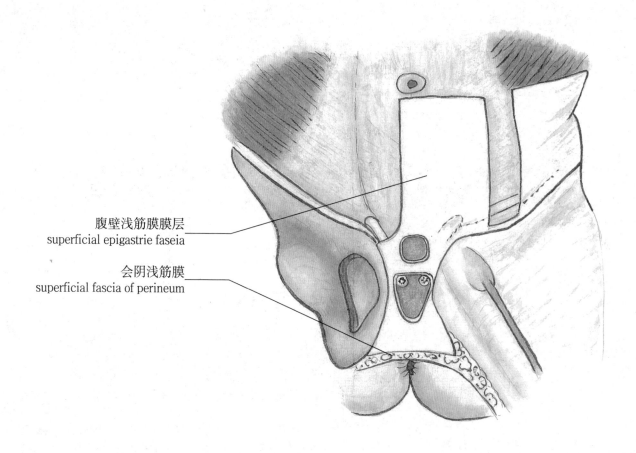

腹壁浅筋膜膜层
superficial epigastrie faseia

会阴浅筋膜
superficial fascia of perineum

图 8-19　男性会阴浅筋膜
Superficial faseia of perineum of the man

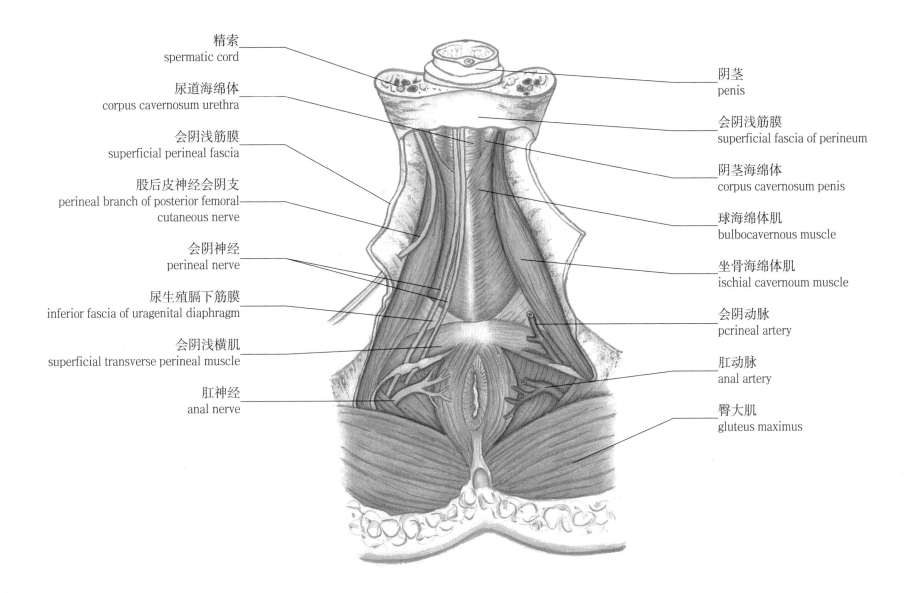

精索
spermatic cord

尿道海绵体
corpus cavernosum urethra

会阴浅筋膜
superficial perineal fascia

股后皮神经会阴支
perineal branch of posterior femoral
cutaneous nerve

会阴神经
perineal nerve

尿生殖膈下筋膜
inferior fascia of uragenital diaphragm

会阴浅横肌
superficial transverse perineal muscle

肛神经
anal nerve

阴茎
penis

会阴浅筋膜
superficial fascia of perineum

阴茎海绵体
corpus cavernosum penis

球海绵体肌
bulbocavernous muscle

坐骨海绵体肌
ischial cavernoum muscle

会阴动脉
pcrineal artery

肛动脉
anal artery

臀大肌
gluteus maximus

图 8-20　男性会阴浅隙的结构
Superficial perineal spale of male

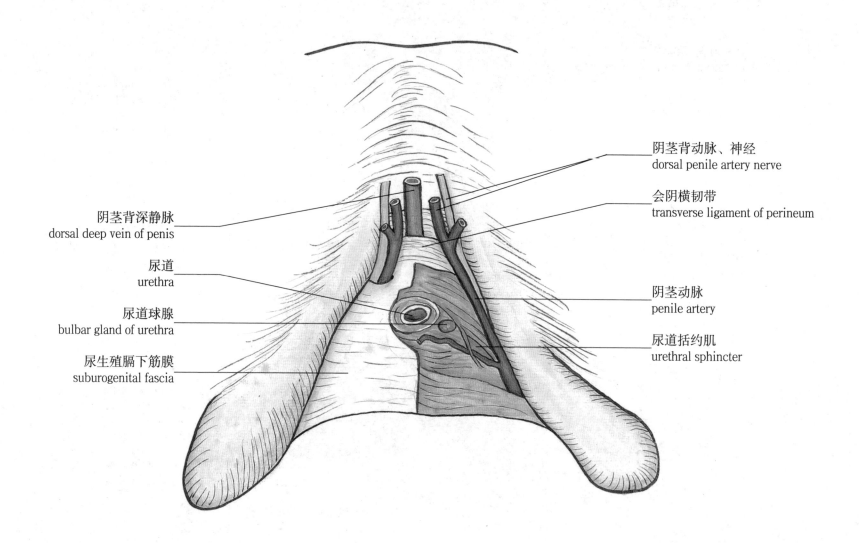

阴茎背动脉、神经
dorsal penile artery nerve

会阴横韧带
transverse ligament of perineum

阴茎背深静脉
dorsal deep vein of penis

尿道
urethra

尿道球腺
bulbar gland of urethra

尿生殖膈下筋膜
suburogenital fascia

阴茎动脉
penile artery

尿道括约肌
urethral sphincter

图 8-21　男性会阴深隙的结构
Deep perineal space of male

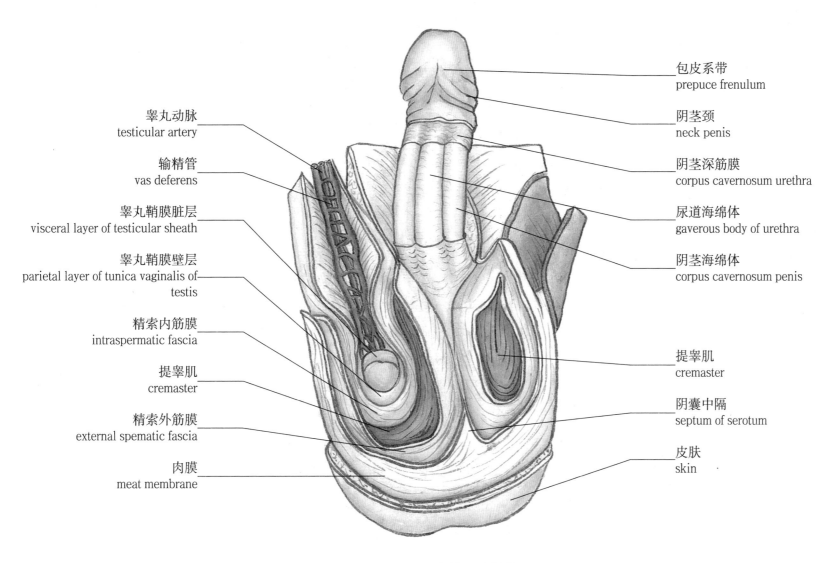

睾丸动脉
testicular artery

输精管
vas deferens

睾丸鞘膜脏层
visceral layer of testicular sheath

睾丸鞘膜壁层
parietal layer of tunica vaginalis of testis

精索内筋膜
intraspermatic fascia

提睾肌
cremaster

精索外筋膜
external spematic fascia

肉膜
meat membrane

包皮系带
prepuce frenulum

阴茎颈
neck penis

阴茎深筋膜
corpus cavernosum urethra

尿道海绵体
gaverous body of urethra

阴茎海绵体
corpus cavernosum penis

提睾肌
cremaster

阴囊中隔
septum of serotum

皮肤
skin

图 8-22　阴囊的层次结构
The level of scrotum

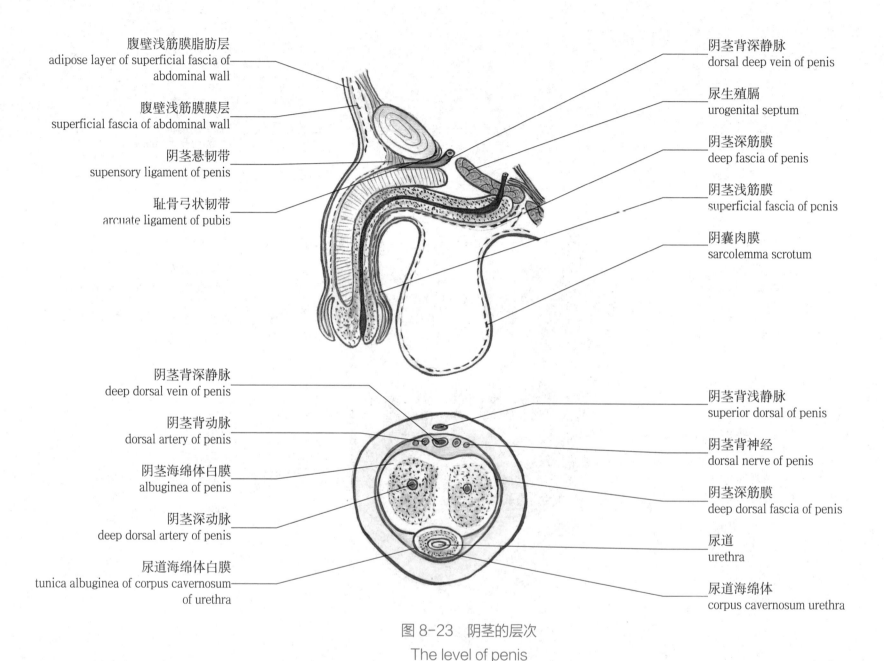

腹壁浅筋膜脂肪层
adipose layer of superficial fascia of
abdominal wall

腹壁浅筋膜膜层
superficial fascia of abdominal wall

阴茎悬韧带
supensory ligament of penis

耻骨弓状韧带
arcuate ligament of pubis

阴茎背深静脉
dorsal deep vein of penis

尿生殖膈
urogenital septum

阴茎深筋膜
deep fascia of penis

阴茎浅筋膜
superficial fascia of penis

阴囊肉膜
sarcolemma scrotum

阴茎背深静脉
deep dorsal vein of penis

阴茎背动脉
dorsal artery of penis

阴茎海绵体白膜
albuginea of penis

阴茎深动脉
deep dorsal artery of penis

尿道海绵体白膜
tunica albuginea of corpus cavernosum
of urethra

阴茎背浅静脉
superior dorsal of penis

阴茎背神经
dorsal nerve of penis

阴茎深筋膜
deep dorsal fascia of penis

尿道
urethra

尿道海绵体
corpus cavernosum urethra

图 8-23　阴茎的层次
The level of penis

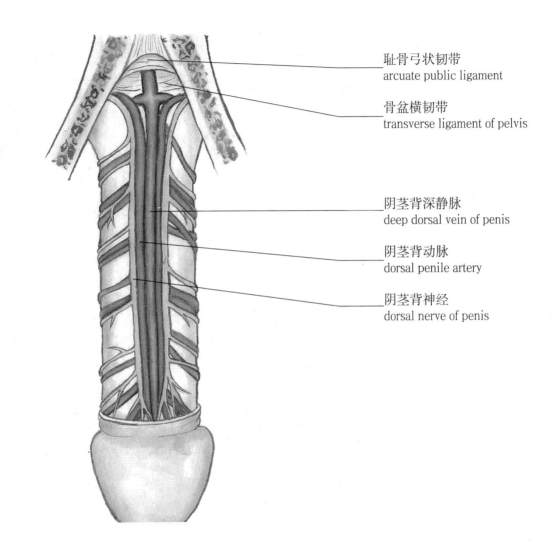

耻骨弓状韧带
arcuate public ligament

骨盆横韧带
transverse ligament of pelvis

阴茎背深静脉
deep dorsal vein of penis

阴茎背动脉
dorsal penile artery

阴茎背神经
dorsal nerve of penis

图 8-24　阴茎背血管和神经
Dorsal blood vessel and nerve of penis

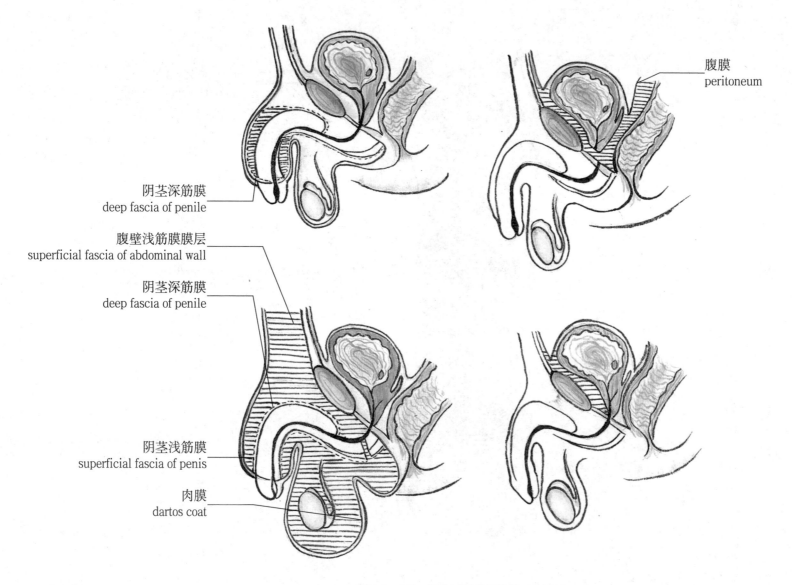

阴茎深筋膜
deep fascia of penile

腹壁浅筋膜膜层
superficial fascia of abdominal wall

阴茎深筋膜
deep fascia of penile

阴茎浅筋膜
superficial fascia of penis

肉膜
dartos coat

腹膜
peritoneum

图 8-25　男性尿道损伤与尿外渗
The damage of urethra and extravasation of urine